The Book About Getting Older

The Book About Getting Older

(for people who don't want to talk about it)

DR LUCY POLLOCK

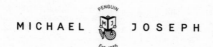

MICHAEL JOSEPH

MICHAEL JOSEPH

UK | USA | Canada | Ireland | Australia
India | New Zealand | South Africa

Michael Joseph is part of the Penguin Random House group of companies
whose addresses can be found at global.penguinrandomhouse.com

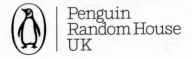

First published by Michael Joseph, 2021

002

Copyright © Lucy Pollock, 2021

The moral right of the author has been asserted

Set in 13.5/16 pt Garamond MT Std
Typeset by Jouve (UK), Milton Keynes
Printed and bound in Great Britain by Clays Ltd, Elcograf S.p.A.

The authorized representative in the EEA is Penguin Random House Ireland,
Morrison Chambers, 32 Nassau Street, Dublin D02 YH68

A CIP catalogue record for this book is available from the British Library

ISBN: 978–0–241–42339–4

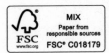

In memory of Anthony Pollock

Contents

CONTENTS

Prologue

In February 2020 I sat at my desk wondering how to indicate a task completed. I had written the last chapter of a book that I had wanted to write for decades, which might help my patients, and those who love them – which might perhaps help all of us as we envisage a future that includes years of life far beyond those of previous generations.

I typed 'the end' in a variety of fonts, but none seemed satisfactory. If I had done my job properly, I had reached not the end of a book but the beginning of a conversation.

Less than a year later, it feels as if coronavirus has changed everything. It has changed how we live, and with whom. It has changed where we work, what we wear, who we see, how we greet one another. It has altered futures, has broken and forged relationships. It has taught us a new and unwelcome vocabulary, of social distancing, shielding and self-isolation. It has brought suffering, loneliness and loss.

Yet the things that mattered most about getting older before COVID-19 still matter most now. Has it become easier to talk about them? For many perhaps not. Fear, urgency and misinformation cloud the picture. Has the conversation become more important? Of course. Now, more than ever, the time has come to tread carefully, to treat one another with kindness and respect, and to speak honestly, gently, clearly. We need to work out how to talk about delicate subjects. We need to explore how the shape of our society might be altered, to make the most of the opportunities granted by long lives. We need to consider how we can work together to create a path that allows us to walk into our future, getting older with confidence, sure-footed.

Author's Note

The people in this book – older people, their families, friends and carers – seem very real to me. I can picture their mannerisms, clothes, expressions. I can see an emerald ring, a stripy tie, a creased handbag, can feel a tremor, hear a phrase or a laugh. And yet none of them are real – they are woven together from multiple tiny threads of reality drawn individually from the cloth of others' lives. Each person is imagined, with imagined experiences, hopes and worries, but I hope that they will seem solid and truthful, for each has a story to tell. My colleagues, however, are entirely real. I have changed their names to spare their blushes.

1. How to be Old

It is your birthday. You are about to blow out the candles on your cake, when you realize that for the first time in your life your chance of living until your next birthday is less than fifty-fifty. What age might you be when this happens? At what age do you develop a less than even chance of living another year?

When I ask my medical students this question they start guessing. Seventy? (The students are very young, and I correct them with a raised eyebrow.) Eighty-one, they venture, knowing that this is the average life expectancy in the UK. I push them upwards. The figure is derived from UK census data, averaged across men and women. Let's put the question another way: if we had a party of ninety-year-olds, would we expect half to have died by next year? Frowning, they guess again, but none get the answer.

It is 104.

Late one night in a hospital in London in 1995, I had just seen Mrs Mildmay. I was the medical registrar on call, and she had been admitted earlier that week with a bad cough and worsening confusion. Despite antibiotics and intravenous fluids, her blood pressure was dropping.

1

Her kidneys had stopped working, and her oxygen level was stubbornly refusing to come up. In her late eighties, she had dementia, and she had been living alone since the death of her husband a few years previously.

I sat with her son John. 'I'm so sorry . . . she seems comfortable, and I think she's peaceful, but it doesn't look as if our treatment is working. It's a really bad pneumonia, and I think she's going to slip away.'

He looked stricken. I put my hand on his arm. His head was bowed, his shoulders hunched.

'Sorry, doctor. It's just – well, Dad died of heart failure and diabetes. And now Mum's got dementia and pneumonia. I wouldn't mind if it was natural causes, but all these diseases really get me down.'

At the time I couldn't help a smile. What, I wondered, did John think old people died of? What would 'natural causes' be, if not pneumonia or heart failure? It has taken me another twenty-five years of looking after very old people and their families, to work out what John was talking about.

We live a long time in the UK – vaccinated, well nourished, provided with clean water, and free from war and violence, we are protected from the scourges that carried off our ancestors prematurely in the past.* That

---

* Even now, with coronavirus whipping its way around the world, we must hold two thoughts simultaneously: that although most people who die of COVID-19 are older, at the same time most older people who get coronavirus (even in their eighties and nineties) will not die of it. Many older people who get infected do not even become seriously

special age of 104, used to grab the attention of medical students, is real. Even though it's a bit of a statistical trick (it doesn't mean half of all people will live to be 104 – very few achieve that), it reminds us that we can reasonably expect a very long life. Only four in one hundred people celebrating their eightieth birthday will die before they turn eighty-one. In 2018 the age at which British women most commonly died was eighty-nine; for men the favourite age of departure was eighty-six.

Increases in life expectancy are greeted with enthusiasm by public health experts, because these figures really tell us something about the health of the whole nation; we cannot expect more people to live beyond ninety if we haven't made some progress in improving health at sixty, and at keeping eighty-year-olds well. Some years ago the UK government announced a target that southwest England should have the highest life expectancy of any comparably sized region in Europe, and by 2013 we had achieved that.

Yet when I mention these figures to friends, especially to those who are older, they don't look especially happy. There's a frown, a look of concern. My friend Vivienne, eighty-one and in cheerful good health, asks 'Why would I want to be a hundred? It sounds grim.' There is a frisson of fear that often comes with contemplating extreme old age. The possibilities of pain,

---

unwell. For all its terrifying statistics and heartbreaking individual deaths, this virus does not significantly dent our collective longevity.

loneliness and – most of all – loss of independence are unwelcome spectres that hover beside us while Vivienne and I talk.

The goalposts of life expectancy have moved. When I was a newly qualified doctor in 1990 none of the hospital patients I looked after were a hundred years old. Centenarians were rare; they lived, were celebrated, and died, in nursing homes. A few years later, the occasional hundred-year-old lady was sent in by a keen GP, but she invariably died in hospital. In the 2000s there were more: some were still living in their own homes, and a few fared a little better – they survived the hospital admission, but didn't recover well enough to get home again and had to move into care. But the posts keep moving. Last winter we looked after Dora who had been admitted after a fall. She stayed a few days to get over an infection, then returned to her bungalow aged 108. Samuel, and Mrs Wilkins, aged 104 and 103, both went home from our ward. As Age UK describes them, older people in this country are 'spirited and resilient'. There are splendid nonagenarians who lead lives of great productivity or contented reflection. Multitudes of older people are loved and supported by devoted partners and families, or live in care homes where, as a patient's daughter Joanne said of her dad's team 'the staff are like angels – they fly to him'. Older people for whom daily survival looks almost impossible often judge their own quality of life much more favourably than the younger onlooker would guess.

But we need to be honest too; being very old is hard work. Lots of difficult and sad things happen, and many old people are not happy. Their families and carers are often exhausted, worried and angry. Being very old has always been a challenge – even when 'very old' was seventy. However, something has changed. Over the years there have been huge advances in medicine, especially in the treatment of the big killers like heart attacks and cancer. Pneumonia, called the 'Captain of the Men of Death' by the physician William Osler a century ago, is kept at bay in all but the most severe cases. However, to our shame, we have not made similar advances in those conditions that cause disability. Bog-standard osteoarthritis and back pain. Intractable itchy skin and tedious leg ulcers. Embarrassing continence problems. Recurrent seemingly minor infections that a younger person would shrug off, but which completely derail the vulnerable older person. Fatigue, and falls, and fear of falls. And, of course, the big D – dementia with its inexorably cruel progress.

Across Europe governments have been measuring not only life expectancy but also 'healthy life expectancy', or similar measures of how long we can expect to live independently and free from disability. In many countries, including the UK, disability-free life expectancy has increased – but it hasn't increased as much as overall life expectancy. The result is that we are living longer *with* disability. Indeed, the figures may be painting a rather rosier picture than they might. Disability is generally measured in terms of whether a person can complete certain day-to-day tasks, and two major technological innovations of the late twentieth century have revolutionized our ability to carry out some of the things we need to do to live independently. These innovations aren't especially glamorous, being simply the shower and the microwave oven, but it's easy to see how they both give someone a better chance of managing without help. So more people are living longer with disability, *and* more people who would previously have been counted as disabled are now reclassified as 'disability-free'. However we cut it, life in old age would appear to have become more difficult for many people. Dodging the conditions that kill us means we must live with those that make life hard.

For nearly thirty years I have been learning from very old people. All geriatricians are asked, 'Don't you find it depressing?' We are told, 'I couldn't do your job'. But I love my job. I've loved it from the moment when I was a very junior doctor and a sensible consultant told me he hoped I wouldn't be offended but he thought I should do geriatric medicine. Immediately I knew he was right, because old people are interesting. And they are also boring, and good-humoured, and bad-tempered. They are serene and irritable. They're amusing and grouchy, selfish and generous, happy-go-lucky and nervy. They're demanding and grateful. They have warm happy families, and terrible angry families, and no families at all.

They have cats and dogs, birds and horses, and boy-friends, and model railways, and houses in Minorca. They've drawn maps and fought in wars and mopped floors, and dug up archaeology, and emptied dustbins, and fostered children. And older people have compli-cated things wrong with them, with multiple illnesses, and a swirl of medications competing for attention, and strange blood and X-ray results that may or may not matter, so it's a real challenge getting the art of medicine right. And each of them has his or her own expect-ations, hopes and fears, and they may or may not be ready or able to tell me what those are. And very old people are supremely vulnerable, and it's immensely easy to make things worse instead of better. Why wouldn't you want to be a geriatrician?

Happily this passion for tackling the complicated stuff is shared by an increasing number of doctors. Early in my career I listened to the pioneers of geriatric medicine as they confronted ageism and established a scientific evidence basis for our work. More recently I've been watching with delight as young trainees find out what's irresistible about 'gerries', and I've seen my own depart-ment blossom and grow. What is it that captivates these doctors, who are still in their twenties when they choose to train in this specialty? For me, and I suspect for many of them too, it's the combination of complex science and unpredictable humanity that appeals. We like working out what the blood results might mean, and looking at the research behind a treatment recommendation – but we love too hearing about the grandchild, or the farm, or the good husband who died. An inspiring colleague, Lindsey, told me years ago, 'You have to be really nosy to be a good geriatrician.' We like being finickety about details ('Precisely how low is his sodium level – just a bit, or enough to explain what's happening?'); we try to be good detectives ('When exactly was this newly confused lady given that particular medication among the thirteen others she's taking?'); we are happy when we feel we've seen the whole picture ('I've realized that Mr Hardy can't make a decision until *Test Match Special* is over'); and we love getting indignant on behalf of our patients ('They can't refuse her an angio just because she's ninety-three!').

Alongside medics who have become interested in looking after the very old, there's a growing cohort of other professionals – nurses, physios and occupational therapists, hospital managers, social workers and care home staff, pharmacists and research scientists – who have made it their business to work out how to make life better in old age. I have had the good fortune to meet therapists who can divine precisely what unspoken fear is preventing my patient from taking her next step, and care home staff who scatter rose petals in the empty room of their resident on the day of her funeral. I've learned about the application of science, and about the medical care of people who have a dozen different diseases at once, and about bizarre drug interactions. I've learned unexpected things: that people who have

Parkinson's disease not only have a different sense of smell but also smell subtly different, and that putting a potato under your pillow might (or might not) help ward off cramp. I've learned how the Mental Capacity Act works when someone has such bad dementia that she can't remember anything except that she is never, ever going to agree to go into a care home. I've learned as I've watched people care for their partners and parents, and for complete strangers, with exasperation, tenderness and love. I've learned that we shy away from conversations we ought to have, and I've learned that everything gets better if we can bring ourselves to have those conversations. Most of all I've learned that we don't talk enough about what it is like to be very old, and I hope this book may help change that.

Older people are just all of us grown up. The huge leap in longevity of the last hundred years offers us unprecedented opportunities – better health, increased independence, more time on this unique planet. Yet sometimes it feels as if things have moved too fast – we are unsettled by this change in the shape of a human life. We haven't worked out yet what we want from our new long lives, or how to develop the kind of society – interconnected, optimistic, fair – that can offer the best chance of delivering well-being and fulfilment to all of us at every age. We haven't even worked out what words to use: 'elderly' as a collective noun ('the elderly') has been consigned to the bin, although some Americans like 'elderhood'; we must tiptoe gingerly around 'frail', being aware that words matter and that it's easy to reinforce the wrong stereotypes, because by no means are all older people frail, and yet we must acknowledge the challenges for those who are. My own professional association, the British Geriatrics Society, ties itself in knots every few years, as it reconsiders its own name, simultaneously shamed by the negative connotations of the word 'geriatric', yet proud of this specialty, this inclusive, multi-professional discipline that demands that we pay attention not only to medical fact but to the entire shape and meaning of a life.

This book is for anyone who is living with some of the problems my patients have. It's for people who are getting very old, and for those who love them. It's for all of us, who will, if we are lucky, become old. It's about what I have learned from skilled, kind colleagues, from families and from my inimitable patients, about how to ask delicate questions, and what to do with the answers, and what to do when the going gets tough – it explains what I have learned about how to be old.

I was driving to work one morning when I heard a gardener talking on the radio about a new caterpillar species attacking nursery plants. I could hear his smile as he said, 'You know how it is. Where there's life, there's trouble.' I love trouble. Let's go.

2. The Big Questions

Irene and I have been talking about her treatment – or, rather, I've been doing most of the talking, and Irene has nodded politely, agreeing with my plan to treat her chest infection and get her out of bed and back home again as soon as possible. She's had a cough for a few days and has become very wobbly on her feet – yesterday she was on her way to her kitchen to make supper when her legs 'just gave out' and she sank to the floor. Her heart's not perfect either. If she doesn't take a couple of water tablets each day, she gets breathless and her ankles puff up. She's told me how tired she feels all the time. 'Just . . . this sounds silly, but I look at the butter dish when it's empty and I think, *Do I have the strength to wash that dish or shall I just put the new butter in?*' And she's had a couple of tumbles before now. Last year she broke her hip doing no more than pulling on her freezer door. It opened with a pop and she fell backwards.

'I think you're going to feel better tomorrow,' I say.

Irene glances at me, then looks out of the window.

I feel bad: my platitude may be true, but it doesn't mean she's ever going to feel properly well again, and Irene knows that. She's already on the best available treatment for her dodgy heart, and I don't have a pill that's going to restore her vitality.

'I'm sorry. You must be feeling a bit downhearted,' I say as I slip my hand under her fingers; the cannula that is used to deliver antibiotics into her blood is dangling precariously on the back of her wrist, and her thin skin is blooming with purple bruises. But her nails are neatly polished, and her wedding and engagement rings shine where they sit loosely between her knobbly joints. Her hair has been recently silvered and set. 'Um . . . Mrs Walton, Irene, do you mind me asking something?'

She turns to me again, and frowns a little as she nods.

I go on. 'Are there times when you go to bed at night and you wish you just wouldn't wake up in the morning?'

Irene's face breaks into a huge smile. She looks directly at me. 'That's exactly how I feel!'

We are at a point in the history of humanity where more and more people are living to a very great age. But we don't really know how to be that old, and we don't always know the best way to live among and look after people who are that old. We don't know what to think when we are facing the big problems of frailty. It's not a subject any of us want to dwell upon, and when we are forced into a situation where we do have to think about being very old, or when we love someone who is very old, we are at a loss. There are so many questions roiling around, like sea waves pounding into a rocky bay, and we don't know how to talk honestly about them. Are we allowed to ask these questions? Are we even allowed to think them?

This book is about the big questions posed by living to a very old age: what the questions are, how to ask them, and some of the answers. We'll look at what makes it hard to ask some of these questions, and why life can get so much better when we get past the barriers that stop us talking about these things.

Irene and I now start having a proper conversation. I ask her how long she has felt this way – felt that she would like to close her eyes and slip away.

'Oh, about six years maybe. Since my husband died.'

'You must have been married a long time?'

'Fifty-nine years.' She smiles proudly.

'I bet you miss him very much. Was he a nice chap?'

'Oh, he was the best!'

We talk about where she met him, at a dance just after the war. She tells me about their travels when he was still in the navy, and his kindness. I ask Irene to tell me what makes her smile. She loves seeing her daughters who live locally and pop in most days, and her son comes down from Kent sometimes, and she enjoys visits from her grandson and his fiancée. She sleeps well ('Too well really, half the day as well') and eats enough. She treats herself to a thimbleful of sherry at six thirty every day. Irene's absolutely clear that she's not depressed. 'I've just had enough. I've had a nice life and I'm tired. I want to be with Tom.'

I ask Irene if there was a tablet that would just end it all, would she take it?

'Oh no,' she tells me, looking quite cross that I have suggested such a thing. 'I wouldn't do that; my family would be upset and it's wrong anyway. No, I can wait my time. But . . . well . . . every night I get into bed and I blow a little kiss to all my children and I hope I'll just . . . you know . . .' She flutters her fingers.

Everything about our conversation is more cheerful now. We've got one of the big questions out of the way – it feels as if she and I have pulled it like a parcel out of her overnight bag, unwrapped it and laid it on the blanket between us, where we can both see it. Now we can talk about whether Irene really is going to recover and get home – I think she will, and we'll give it our best shot. The physio is going to see her this afternoon. But you can never be sure treatments are going to work when you're ninety-two. We discuss what we should do if she gets worse. We agree that whatever happens she doesn't want to go to the intensive care unit (ICU). We decide together that we'll see how she gets on with the intravenous antibiotics, and if she's getting better, that's good, and we'll keep going, but if she's deteriorating, we will stop the treatments that are aimed at keeping her alive, which means, I explain, that she would not get better, that she would spend longer and longer asleep, and that at some point she would gently stop breathing and would not wake up again.

Asking the big questions (one of which is 'Do you

actually want to be alive any more?', although there are more sensitive ways of asking that, which I'll come to) allows the rest of the conversation to become more honest. Irene's concerns, which we have unpacked together, are about what has meaning for her, and what her future holds, and what control she might have over that future. It's important that she is given space to talk about these things. If she and I do not have that conversation right now, and she becomes less well, decisions may be taken that do not reflect her wishes.

Cathy, one of Irene's daughters, arrives just as I'm leaving.

'Do you mind if I explain to Cathy what we were talking about?' I ask.

Irene nods and I talk about the decisions we've made.

'I'm not surprised you said that,' says Cathy, who is wearing a pink fluffy jumper and has a gentle face. She looks like her mother: her bright eyes are the same, with the wrinkles born of smiles rather than frowns. Cathy pats Irene's hand.

'You've wanted to be with Dad since the day he died really, haven't you, Mum? We all understand that.'

I'm glad Cathy knows now what her mum's wishes are. Irene clearly is able to make her own decisions, and legally there's no real need to share with her family the conversation she and I have had. But if she gets too unwell to speak, or becomes confused (which might easily happen, because even the sparkiest older brain is vulnerable), Cathy and the rest of Irene's family will be asked to help with decisions about what level of treatment Irene would want: things like being fed by tube, or using a machine to help with her breathing. Without having talked to her mum about these things Cathy may well be able to guess at Irene's wishes, but it's likely that she'll feel responsible for deciding whether treatment should be continued or stopped. Frankly, however delicately the doctors put it, Cathy may be presented with a situation in which her words will seem to make the difference in deciding whether her mother lives or dies. From talking to families caught in situations like this I know those conversations are never forgotten and hang heavily on each conscience. If we tackle the questions more openly, that doesn't have to happen. And the questions aren't just about what happens at the end, about dying – they are about the problems that arise while we *live* in old age.

Here are some of the big unspoken questions: How do I know if someone's getting dementia? How do I know if *I* am getting dementia? How do I decide whether to have that operation? Are these tablets worth taking? What'll happen if my mum doesn't take her medicines? Am I going to have to go into a home, and if I do, will it be awful? Should Mum go into a home, and if she doesn't, how guilty will I feel if she breaks her hip falling down stairs? Are the doctors going to try hard enough to keep Dad alive? Or are they going to try too hard? Am I truthfully still safe to drive? What words should I use when I'm trying to talk to a nurse about Dad's . . .

gentleman parts? How do I ask a doctor whether it would be OK not to treat my husband's pneumonia? If I ask that question, will people think I don't love him? What do doctors have to do – what does the Hippocratic oath mean anyway? Are doctors allowed to not treat someone, or is that euthanasia? How do I talk to someone about my fear of dying? Or is it OK that I wish to be dead? Yet more difficult, is it OK to say – am I allowed even to feel – that I wish for the death of someone that I truly love?

These are questions that we feel unable to ask. They become worries because we can't have an honest conversation about them. They are worries that keep my eighty-nine-year-old aunt awake at night. They are worries that a daughter churns over on her way to work, that an elderly husband can't share with his wife. They are worries a son has when he's running a business in Turkey and his mum is in her assisted-living flat in Ramsgate. And every single one of these questions creates more questions that we should ask, should talk about, and should be able to share.

There are plenty more. Is it OK to admit that I am repelled by old age? That I cannot cope with the idea of incontinence? How do I tell someone, anyone, that my dearly beloved husband of almost sixty years has been talking about *sex* to young carers? Every question that you can think of, everything you feel you can't say, is a question that someone else has worried about too, and is one that needs to be asked.

One of my favourite cartoons features a very large elephant sitting glumly in the dock of a courtroom. He's being harangued by a lawyer, who says, 'If you were in the room the whole time, how come we cannot find a single witness to corroborate your story?' As we each explore the new, unfamiliar world of very old age, great herds of elephants are clumping around in every room, and we have got to work out ways to talk about them. What are the barriers that make us unable to ask the most important questions?

One summer day, years ago, I had collected the children from school. They were small and were hot and sticky in the back of the car. We stopped at temporary traffic lights in a village on the way home, and I could see a very old woman coming along the pavement towards us. She was moving slowly, using a walking frame. Her body was bent forward and sideways both at once, her left shoulder so low it was almost touching the frame, on which swung a small bag of shopping. Despite the sun she was wearing a felt hat that shaded her face, but as she neared I could see her eyes close just before she lifted the frame. Slow blink . . . lift the frame . . . set it down . . . shuffle forward . . . repeat. On a lead behind her a tiny three-legged terrier skipped merrily about, investigating the delicious scents of wall and gutter. The twisted old woman came slowly closer, and there was a wail from the back seat. 'Mummy, look! Poor little dog!'

Part of the problem is that we choose to make very

old people invisible, and we choose not to hear their voices. This invisibility, these unheard voices, are created and kept in place by three great barriers. The first two are prejudice and fear, which are intertwined. And the third is the biggest of all, but we'll come to that later.

Let's get prejudice out of the way. It seems to have been with us forever; we recognize so easily the ugly old wicked witches of Greek legend and Brothers Grimm fairy tales. Unlikeable old men – stupid, greedy or both – pop up everywhere from Roman farces to the novels of Dickens. Shakespeare is not kind to the old. I'm not sure it's even prejudice; authors and playwrights have been mocking human traits since time began, and are just as ready to dish the dirt on the feckless youth, the overbearing mother and the preposterous tyrant. But maybe if we collectively could look honestly into the heart of our society, we would have to admit that we do regard old people as burdensome.

We do this at a national level, with talk from economists, politicians and journalists referring to the 'burden' of ageing, the 'demographic time bomb', and the 'economically inactive', who raid rather than fatten the national purse. Successive governments have kicked the question of equitable funding for care in old age firmly down the road, and with each kick the impression we are given is that the problem is just too intractable to handle. GCSE geography students are asked not 'what should we welcome about increasing life expectancy?', but rather 'how can we cope with an ageing population?' There is little focus on the positives, such as the economic benefits of grandparents who take on childcare, allowing those of working age to contribute more; the cheerful consumerism of the retired, the volunteering – the charity shops, the local history society, the litter-picking group; the experience and wisdom and love that older relatives can bring, especially to fractured families; the sheer delight of having more years in retirement, freed from the nine-to-five, our time our own. These are the rich dividends of successful ageing, worthy of celebration rather than hand-wringing. We should hang out the bunting for our national longevity!

On an individual level too we all have our prejudices. We are often uneasy about being with the very old. They are different from us, and none of us like difference. We don't like people who talk weirdly, or who might be muddled, because they make us feel awkward or embarrassed. We perhaps worry that old people might be racist, or sexist – and some of them are. Plenty of old people blithely use language that makes the rest of us wince, quite unaware that their words convey views they don't hold; my own stepfather, who in the navy championed the rights of gay men and campaigned for women to be allowed to serve at sea, talks fondly of the 'poofty bag' in which he carries his purse and diary. And old people drive slowly! They take ages to find their change in shops! They use the loo for hours when everyone else is queuing!

And, of course, prejudice lurks in the bushes on the

other side of the age gap too. The young have the vitality, the energy, the spring-out-of-bed, which will never again be accessible to the very old. Jealousy is an undercurrent that hums beneath familiar phrases: 'My daughter's life is so busy'; 'Our neighbours, always rushing here and there'. The young are on their phones all the time. They don't dress properly, and the boys have long hair and the girls have short hair and they're all in a muddle about being gay or lesbian, which wouldn't matter if only they'd make their minds up. And they slouch and mumble, and use terrible language, and don't make eye contact. They don't write thank-you letters, and they can't cook, and they don't go to church. Small wonder we have some communication problems.

The next barrier that gets in the way of our conversations is fear. Again, this plays out on both large and small scales. Nationally there's a fear that caring for the very old will prove our economic undoing, or at least our political nemesis. Governments fear that whatever social care funding mechanism they propose, the backlash will be severe from those who feel most hard done by. Political heads will roll, votes will be lost and parties ousted from power. Better to bury the Dilnot report on the funding of care and support, delay the White Paper, abandon the 'dementia tax'.

For each of us in our individual relationships fear hangs around unacknowledged. Being with very old people may mean having to deal with physical problems that we don't want to contemplate. We have to confront bristly nostrils and whiskery chins, and help put socks on gnarled feet, and buy Marigold gloves. I recall with shame the first time I peered into a very old man's mouth as a medical student. The sight caused me visibly to recoil, and if I'm truthful, I made a retchy sound too.

Thirty years later, I was giving my younger daughter a lift to school. She was revising for biology GCSE, but was already clear that she had no intention of becoming a doctor. She looked up from the revision quiz on her phone. 'Mum, which one takes the waste products out of the kidney, ureter or urethra?'

I absolutely love this sort of question and launched in.

'OK, darling, it's the ureter. But the urethra is very interesting too, because it's a sort of design fault in women, which is why we get urine infections so easily. The urethra is too short, so bacteria can easily climb up into the bladder, which is why you have to make sure you drink enough, and be careful to finish your pee properly, and always wipe your bottom from front to back. Anyway, how are you going to remember which is which for the exam? Well, there's just one urethra, *a* urethr*a*, and there are two ureters, one for each kidney, so you can think, "t-t-two ure-t-t-ters". Do you think that will help?'

My lovely daughter stared out of the passenger window. 'It's disgusting,' she murmured. 'I'd rather die than remember that.'

I have become hardy about physical imperfection now, but many people just aren't and never will be. Any talk about the workings of the body makes some feel queasy. Unhappy emotions like these not only affect how younger people feel about the aged, but also influence how the very old feel about themselves. This wariness of contemplating unlovely biological detail is not something that necessarily changes with age; my friend's mum Margaret gloomily remarked of her companions, 'We start all our tea parties with an organ recital – which organ has everyone got going wrong this time. It's not my favourite subject.'

In order to talk about some of the difficulties of very old age we have to confront bodily problems that repel us, and for many that takes courage. And, of course, there is fear of the future, where the very old see only death. For some that prospect is filled with horror: gazing into the abyss. For others, like my dear aunt, the fear is of loss of independence. 'I'm fine as I am now,' she says, 'and I'm not worried about what happens after I die. It's the grey area in between . . .' She shivers.

I was leaning on the bar in Jonny O's pub in the west of Ireland, having a moan to Maureen the landlady. Mum had been on the phone, wanting to know when we would be back from holiday, so that the children would do her online order for a new senior railcard, and I would be able to referee her current dispute with the Royal Albert Hall, and my husband would design and build a reflective panel to sit behind one of her radiators, the better to direct more heat into her already sweltering kitchen. I explained this to Maureen, who rubbed a glass with a cloth and said comfortably, 'Well, my children say to me, "Mother, we will not hear you say a bad word about Nanna, because, sure, she's the way you are going."'

Steady on, Maureen! You haven't met my mum! But her words – or rather her children's words – stayed with me. I have to think about my mum and the things she does that I love, and the things she does that I really don't love. I recognize patterns that run through us both like a stick of rock, and it's not a comfortable process. Our parents and grandparents look at us, and their faces say, 'Here I am, your future,' and that can make us afraid.

When I asked an older geriatrician, Sammy, about how we might encourage people to talk about the big questions of ageing, he was worried.

'I don't think geriatricians can be part of this project,' he said. 'It looks too . . .' His voice trailed off.

'Too what?' I niggled.

Sammy is a fantastic doctor. His ability to have sensitive conversations that make people feel better is second to none. Why would he think we should not be part of a movement that encourages openness and helps people get to grips with these important problems?

Sammy looked uncertain. 'I think . . . people will think we're trying to encourage them to give up. It might mean they lose confidence in us. They might think we're not on their side any more.'

Sammy's view filled me with dismay. Geriatricians have conversations with families and patients almost every day. For almost thirty years I've had the privilege of participating in precious, intimate discussions about what matters most with thousands of older people and those who love them. Why would it not be a good idea to share what Sammy and I have learned?

I realized then that this is where fear and prejudice come together in a toxic mix that kills conversations. We don't talk about important things because we fear that people will consider us prejudiced or selfish. A devoted wife may fear that talking with her adult children about the possibility of their father going into care will be perceived as being motivated by a desire to lessen her own burden. Sammy fears that a call from geriatricians for better advance care planning will be interpreted as a wish to reduce demand on our Emergency Departments and wards. We all fear that if we talk about the difficulties of ageing, people will see straight through us and perceive a greedy, mean core within. Prejudice and fear cause us to duck away from important conversations, and fear of being thought to be prejudiced often means we can't tackle the big questions at all. But we need to work out how to talk about them. Having looked after very old people and their families over many years, I know that when these questions are kept locked away they weigh us down with unhappiness, anxiety and anger. Bring them into the light instead, and we can discover reassurance and new-found confidence.

We need to be honest. I will describe how we work out what's treatable, and I'll talk about survival, and recovery, and the practical things people can do to make things happier in very old age, but I am also going to talk about making decisions not to continue treatment, about stopping medications, and about recognizing futility. I will explain what the law says. I'll talk about the ethical principles that guide us, and about how older people and their families can find the words to talk openly with medical teams about their concerns and their hopes. I'll explain how we can work together as a society to remove decisions that are currently driven by stress, emergency and fear, and replace them instead with social structures founded in empathy, ingenuity, energy and a passion for fairness.

I've had to confront my own prejudices again and again.

It had been another hopelessly busy day in the hospital and was shaping up for a horrible night; we medical registrars worked a twenty-four-hour shift and took all the phone calls from GPs and the Accident and Emergency Department about people who needed assessment, at the same time as seeing those who had already arrived: one with maybe meningitis, another with a stroke; a pointless resus attempt for a middle-aged drug user, who had clearly been dead for hours; people with falls, and breathlessness, and chest pain that might be indigestion or might be a catastrophic dissecting aortic aneurysm. By 9 p.m. there were no beds left, and patients were being stacked on trolleys in A & E. My bleep had been pinging incessantly for hours, and I took yet another call. A GP was phoning from a care home to explain that he was sending in a young woman, nineteen years old, with a blocked PEG* feeding tube. 'She's got severe cerebral palsy, unable to communicate, doubly incontinent, full nursing care. Unsafe swallow, can't drink, hasn't had anything through the tube for twenty-four hours. Sorry about that; she's on her way.' I put the phone down and leaned against one of the concrete pillars that stood in the way of every trolley coming into the ward. My thoughts ran on a single miserable theme: *What is the point? What is the point? Why am I wasting my time trying to keep alive someone whose quality of life is so . . . shit?* The bleep pinged again, and I forgot about her.

Hours later, A & E rang. 'Your PEG girl is here.'

I stomped down from the wards and jerked back the cubicle curtain. She sat perched on the trolley. Tiny stick-like contorted black limbs, like a scrappy crow's nest. A little torso no bigger than a six-year-old child's. And her head – her face! – a grin as wide as the sea, and her brown eyes shining with delight.

Right then I swore I would never, ever again make a judgement about someone's quality of life (their life, their right to life), based on what I knew of their

---

* A PEG feeding tube is a percutaneous endoscopic gastrostomy tube, which is inserted through the skin just below the ribs to allow feeding directly into the stomach for someone who can't swallow.

intellectual or physical function. Or, as it happens, their age. Over the years I've seen repeatedly how easy it is for any of us – medical teams, carers, families, me – to jump to conclusions about somebody else's contentment, their hopes or wishes. Prejudice exists, so we have to seek it out in ourselves, and become fearless about acknowledging it. Only then can we do our best to have honest conversations that allow the people to tell us – or show us – what is important to them.

The conversations between very old people and those they love, and the social constructs that dictate how we collectively treat older people, are thus constrained and hampered by fences made of prejudice and fear, but if we can identify these fences, we can find ways past them. Later, I'll look at some of the ways in which we can skirt round these wiry obstacles. But there is one final huge barrier, perhaps the biggest of the three.

George was very ill; he'd been brought in from a residential home where he'd been living for a few years. The care home staff had sent a record of his medications: three pages of computer print-out, eleven different medicines given at four different times of day. His blood pressure was slipping downwards despite bags of intravenous fluids; his fingers were blue, his nose icy cold. He'd had strong antibiotics and was on high-flow oxygen.

I rang the next of kin number. George's daughter Nina answered. I described how unwell George was, and what we had done so far.

'I wish I was with him,' she said, and explained that she was visiting her daughter and the just-born first grandchild miles away in Lancashire.

'Don't feel bad, Nina. I don't think he's aware of anything and he's comfortable. I just want to be sure we are doing the right thing by him. Um . . . to be honest, whatever we do, I think he's got only a very slim chance of getting through this one, because he's very sick, and I wonder if he would want us to keep trying or whether he'd rather we just concentrate on keeping him peaceful.'

I could hear Nina rummage for a hanky. She blew her nose, and told me, 'The thing is, I think he knew this was coming. I saw him last week and he looked fine, well, as fine as he can, and we talked about this and that, like we always do, and he suddenly said –' Nina paused and was quiet for a few seconds before carrying on. 'He said, "Nina, you're a big girl now . . ." and I could tell it was really hard for him to say it because we never talk about that kind of thing, but then he said, "I think you'll get along all right," and he told me he thought his time was up and he didn't mind that, and he was ready to go.'

Nina and I spoke a bit more. After she had rung off I sat with the phone in my hand for a moment. Eilish, the nurse looking after George, came out of his room. I told her what he had said to Nina.

Eilish's cheeks flushed, and she blinked and fanned her face with the drug chart she was carrying. 'Oh dear . . . sorry . . .' Eilish breathed out slowly. 'Kind man . . .'

Oh, George, you brave man. You got it exactly right. You overcame the great barrier that stops us from talking about the most important things: the barrier that is made of love. How can we talk with the children we love about leaving them? Conversations about dementia, physical indignity, mortal illness, separation – we might be able to cope with these in the abstract, when they're about other people, but when they are about those we love – our friends, our husbands, wives, parents, children – we are undone. The very people we need to talk with are the ones with whom we can't even start the conversation. We need to change that; we can do better. We can't each go on thinking, *I can't talk about this because I love you.* Instead we must say, 'It is *because* I love you that we are going to talk about this.'

3. Squaring the Curve – How to be Amazing

I draw a picture for the three medical students. It's a graph that illustrates the shape of our lives. Up the left side is *independence*, and along the bottom is *age*. I start by drawing a line whizzing up the graph.

'Here are my teenage children,' I explain as I'm drawing it, 'busy learning to drive and working out how to look after their money and becoming able to manage their own lives.' (Up to a point. I have recently seen a text exchange between my husband and our son, who has just left home for university. Dad texts, *Have you sent Mum a birthday card?*

Son: *Gonna do mums card today.*
Pause of several hours, then son texts again.
How do I actually send a card, ie buy stamps and stuff?)

I get back to the graph. 'What most people want is to be one hundred per cent independent, and stay alive and well . . .' I talk while I draw a horizontal line, 'Alive and well, alive and well, alive and well – then dead.'

I drop the line vertically, and add a little cross to show when death happens.

'And in the old days, before vaccines, antibiotics and

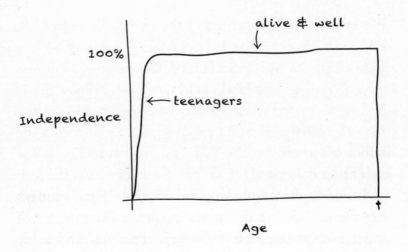

surgery, that's what your life shape looked like. The problem was that the sudden moment of death might happen when you were two, of diphtheria, or fifteen, of typhoid, or twenty-three, by being crushed in a tin mine.' I draw more vertical lines.

'We got good at avoiding those deaths, and we pushed

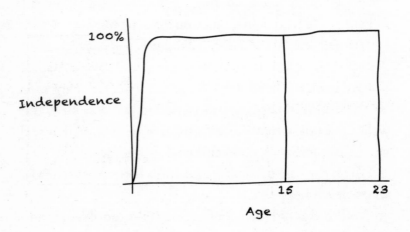

life expectancy further along the graph. But when the end came it generally happened fairly quickly – you didn't last long with cancer before late twentieth-century advances in surgery and chemo, or with kidney failure before dialysis, or with a heart attack before blood thinners and the magic stuff cardiologists do with stents and balloons.'

The students nod.

I redraw the graph on another page. 'Here's today's life shape.' I draw a curve trailing down from the '100% independent' line. 'Here's a wrist fracture, and a hip fracture.' I draw in a couple of jinks. 'A stroke –' the curve jumps down a notch – 'and arthritis and heart failure and dementia. Here you might have moved into a nursing home . . .' The curve is near the bottom now, and wobbles along, before finally meeting the baseline. 'And this is the end.'

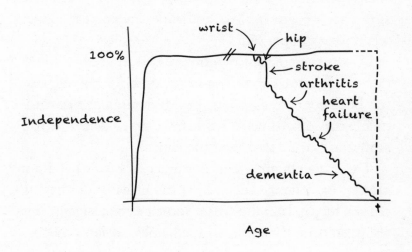

I point to the bottom right-hand corner of the graph, where independence is low and age is high.

'This is where things can be very difficult for people. It isn't difficult for everyone, and it's certainly possible to be happy in this part of the graph, so we can't make judgements about what individuals want without asking them. But having lots of disability, and depending on others for our care, is not what most people want. So overall we agree that there's little point in adding to the life expectancy of the whole population if those extra years are destined to be spent very dependent or in care. We can't just extend life expectancy by adding two more years of being twenty-one.'

The medical students look happy. It's nice being twenty-one.

I set them a problem. 'So the question is, how do we "square the curve"? How do we get rid of the curve of frailty, keep everyone "100% alive and well" and make sure that we are healthy and independent for longer when we are super old?'

This is the concept of 'compressed morbidity' (mortality is dying; morbidity is being unwell). It's one that has been concerning public health doctors and governments for some time. What can we do to delay the bad stuff until we are very near the end?

The students are great, but are not sure what I am asking for. I nudge them: how might we avoid having broken hips in later life? After some hesitant suggestions about starting osteoporosis medicines, which I dismiss as being too little and too late, we talk about what really makes a difference. Starting young! The way to have strong bones in old age is to get those bones as well built as they can be in childhood and adolescence. Running around, and jumping up and down. Playing netball between the ages of fourteen and nineteen when the majority of bone mass is added. (This is one of the reasons why it's criminal that so much new building in cities in the 1980s was on school playing fields.) Later, we can keep our bones as strong as possible by staying active, not smoking, making sure we eat enough calcium, and getting a dose of vitamin D from a few hours each year with our sleeves rolled up in the summer sunshine – not getting sunburned, just modestly shone upon. Osteoporosis medicines may help, but if we have the option, it's got to be better to start off with strong bones in the first place.

In fact, for many conditions we need to start our healthy ageing campaign before we are born – we need a mum who's a sensible weight and doesn't smoke or drink too much, and maybe eats her greens and takes a folic acid tablet each day in early pregnancy, so we start out with the best possible chances. We need to be born healthy. Next, we must collect some childhood vaccinations so that we're not damaged by infectious diseases that sound old-fashioned but haven't gone away. After that, there are some political hard truths. Michael Marmot in *The Health Gap* leads the field on how governments, rather than healthcare organizations, influence life expectancy. A decent education helps – every year spent in full-time learning adds time at the far end of life. Having a job is vitally important. Race, social disadvantage and poverty, horribly intertwined, are scandalously associated with shortened lives. Being rich makes a remarkable difference; life expectancy increases slowly and steadily with every dollar earned, until the top of the scale, where the very richest enjoy a sudden jump in lifespan well above that steady rise. My friend Clodagh is a GP and says, 'What is it with really posh old people? They never die!'

Government policies also influence choices about the things we do when we are young. It helps if laws encourage us not to mess things up in our teens – obviously it's a good idea to avoid dodgy drugs and road accidents that can bring about a neurological catastrophe. Staying off the cigarettes makes a real difference to life expectancy, as does kicking the habit in middle or early old age. Doctors can bang on about these things with some effect, but it is governments that need to legislate on seat belts and cigarette advertising and the quality of school meals.

As we get older the direct effects of healthcare become more influential. Controlling blood pressure and cholesterol levels helps. There's no doubt that hypertension medicines and statins, started for some people in middle age, have contributed to increasing life expectancy. Being treated quickly for a heart attack definitely prevents many premature deaths, and survivors often have a top-notch quality of life. More people now survive cancer. And after emergency treatments, simple medicines like aspirin to render blood less sticky after a heart attack or stroke certainly reduce the chance of another heart attack or stroke. These are 'preventative' medicines, as opposed to the sort that make you feel better, and the story about whether it's worth taking them in super-old age is more controversial – I'll come to that in a later chapter. But a similar conversation needs to take place about what we eat.

I met Leopold some years ago. He was a precise man, a Unitarian preacher, and his wife Mathilde had been in hospital for several months; she had a rare and severe illness, and had been sent from Sussex to London for specialist care. Leopold travelled up two or three times a week to visit her on the ward – a long journey, involving a lift to the station, a train, the tube. He wore a neat dark suit and carried a faded seventies tote bag with a daisy pattern. I watched him unpack it one day: a chocolate cream éclair in a white card box for Mathilde; a tiny bunch of violets in a plastic bag, slightly crushed, their stalks wrapped in wet loo paper; a Bible, with bookmarks and annotated slips of paper poking out. Leopold wobbled as he turned to look for a chair, and I caught his arm, bony through the woollen cloth.

'Mr Trevor, I wonder . . . might you have lost some weight?'

He smiled ruefully. 'Ah, I'm on a bit of a diet.'

'A diet? Why?'

'Well, I had a little touch of angina, and my GP sent me to the cardiologist, and he says my cholesterol is on the high side. He says no cheese or eggs or cream.'

'That sounds a bit fierce!'

'Well, it's a shame, because I really like cheese. But, you know, doctor's orders!'

For a moment I was so cross I wanted to get that cardiologist and hold him by the shoulders and shout, 'Leopold is eighty-six! His wife is mortally unwell! What are you doing?'

In my head my tirade went on: 'How can you possibly suggest that banning foods like that is going to make the slightest difference to what happens next? Show me the evidence for your stupid, pompous, mean-spirited directive! In what way can that make ANYTHING better for this kind, respectful man who will do his utmost to abide by everything you say?'

I busied myself finding a chair for Leopold, went to see some other patients, and let the rage fizzle down. I wanted to protect him from advice that seemed to me to be actively causing him harm, but I didn't want to undermine his faith in his cardiologist. Getting conflicting advice from different doctors is unsettling, especially perhaps for someone like Leopold, with his attention to detail and eagerness to do the right thing – and, in any case, Leopold wasn't my patient. But I was so angry! Later, he came to the desk for an update on Mathilde's progress. I mentioned his own well-being, his loss of weight.

He looked worried. 'You see, I don't want to have a heart attack, because then I won't be able to visit Mathilde. So I am being strict about the diet. What do you think?'

Somehow in his consultation with the cardiologist Leopold had come away with the impression that adherence to this low-fat diet was essential – that a sliver of Brie would bring on crushing central chest pain. That didn't feel fair. I chucked away my professional qualms.

'At this stage I think keeping strong might be the priority. You're working so hard with the long journey . . .'

Leopold waved a thin hand to indicate the unimportance of his travelling time, and raised his eyebrows at me to go on.

'And I think it might be about getting a balance . . . cutting out the cheese and cream and things is likely only to make a very, very small difference to your chance of having a heart attack in the next while. So I think maybe you should allow yourself a sensible amount of cheese.'

He smiled, and patted my arm.

'And, Mr Trevor, Leopold, when you do eat cheese I don't think you should feel guilty, just enjoy it; you're building up your strength to visit Mathilde . . . and that goes for the odd chocolate éclair too.'

*

Our innate longing to control the ageing process leads us to search for the perfect anti-ageing diet, the magical supplement that will prevent dementia, the elixir of youth that might be found in Holland & Barrett or a corner of the internet. But we must brace ourselves for some boring news. The truth is no scientist has ever conclusively proved that one diet or supplement can really improve one's chance of a long and disability-free life. What is the best advice? We can look at the animal-fat-filled 'Western' diet of those who die young, and the 'good' diets of groups of people who seem to last for ages, but it's hard to *prove* that it's the olive oil, the nuts and the high proportion of fruit and vegetables in the Mediterranean diet that actually causes the long life. It's simply difficult to do accurate trials of diets. Researchers can allocate people in a trial to one diet or another, but it's difficult for the participants to stick to a strict diet for the several years necessary to show an effect. And if a participant hears for example that berries might ward off dementia, they might choose to add berries to their diet – which will skew the result if they were part of the group that wasn't meant to be eating berries. So lots of the work about diet is based on observational studies; the researchers just record as accurately as possible what the study participants eat, then see what happens to them. For example, an important study looked at a diet called MIND (Mediterranean-DASH Intervention for Neuro-degenerative Delay), which was created by researchers in

Chicago who wanted to see if it might reduce the risk of dementia.

MIND is a combination of two diets already known to be associated with a reduced risk of heart disease and stroke: the Mediterranean diet (based on whole grains, fish, pulses, fruits and vegetables) and the DASH (Dietary Approaches to Stop Hypertension) diet. The DASH diet is designed to control blood pressure and is similar to the Mediterranean diet, but with a greater emphasis on reducing salt intake. The participants in the MIND study weren't told what to eat, but everything they reported was scored — there were extra marks for the consumption of leafy green vegetables and for berries, because other studies had suggested that these might be associated with better brain function. The results were clear: after almost five years those who stuck most closely to the ideal MIND diet had brains that were the equivalent of 7.5 years younger than those who followed the diet the least. They did better on all the memory tests, and were less likely to have been diagnosed with dementia. However, there were other differences between the groups. Those who stayed closest to the ideal MIND diet were also better educated. They were slightly younger, less obese and less likely to have diabetes at the outset of the study. They started off with lower blood pressures. Overall, the people whose diet was 'best' also started off the most healthy, and were the least likely to get dementia anyway. So the Chicago team had to do some clever statistical tricks to demonstrate that at least part of the reduction in dementia was related to the diet itself, not to other aspects of the participants' lives. The researchers were careful not to overstate their claim. They wrote: 'This prospective study of the MIND diet score provides evidence that greater adherence to the overall dietary pattern may be protective against the development of AD [Alzheimer's disease].' That's a good safe conclusion, and for me it's enough to cause some modifications to my own diet. And there's a positive placebo effect, which is worth embracing: when I eat spinach I feel brainier.

Beyond the clear benefits of a vaguely Mediterranean diet, the arguments about specific foods and supplements will rage on. As I write, eggs are back under scrutiny – for a while eggs were evil: chubby fat-smugglers, furring up arteries with their deposits of cholesterol. Then they got rehabilitated as nutrient-filled protein packages. This week eggs are in the firing line again: once more an observational study suggests that eating lots of eggs may be associated with higher rates of heart disease – but the study didn't look at bacon.

Sadly, because the hard science sends out some conflicting messages, the door is opened to a whole lot of hooey. Claims like 'raspberries contain zeaxanthin, a plant chemical that helps to maintain healthy eyes' are worth being wary of because while that statement may be true it doesn't mean that eating raspberries will do anything for your eyesight. Even worse are statements such as 'hard-core fasting allows the body to repro-gramme itself'. (What does that actually mean? Do I want my body to be 'reprogrammed'?)

An American author, Michael Pollan, has summed up the sensible dietary advice. He uses seven words: 'Eat food, not too much, mostly plants.' By 'eat food' he means unprocessed food – vegetables, fruit, whole grains and small amounts of meat and fish. 'Not too much,' says Pollan; we know obesity is a pervasive threat to a long life – it really does interfere with every-thing, because as well as increasing our risk of cancer, heart disease and diabetes, it makes our knees ache and insidiously slows us down. And 'mostly plants' – the average 'Western' diet contains too much meat, and most people could benefit from swapping more of that meat to grain, pulses, fruit and vegetables. In the end there is an inescapably strong correlation between a long and healthy life and the sort of diet suggested by Pollan, which is the same sort of diet endorsed by the British Heart Foundation, Cancer Research UK and the Alzheimer's Society. Eat your greens. You know it makes sense.

But once you've reached super-old age what then are the rules? Some older people put on weight as they slow down, but for many, as for Leopold, the bigger threat is weight loss. In addition, putting it bluntly, the super-old person may not have time left in which to benefit from the healthy diet. Even those with diabetes have been shown to gain little (perhaps a few weeks of extra life) from a rigid diet and multiple medications to control sugar level when these changes are made after the age of seventy-five. And there may well be so many other things going on that a plateful of curly kale is just a bridge too far.

For the super old all the rules of healthy living are there to be broken. Except perhaps one. I asked Geoffrey, who was ninety-three and had worked as a land agent, how he looked so well. He thought for a while before giving a textbook answer. 'I never smoked; I drank in moderation, worked outdoors and kept active. We grew and ate all our own vegetables. And I married a good woman.' He was right on every count, even down to his marital status: married men do last longer than single ones. The opposite is true for women, but that's more to do with the historical threats posed to women by childbirth, rather than simply being driven to an early grave by the frustration of sharing one's life with a husband. Probably. But Geoffrey's answer contains the secret to a healthy as well as a long life. He kept active.

In 2005 a team of Australian researchers started to look at the walking patterns of a group of men all aged seventy or more. The group was large, 1,705 men from Sydney, and the team measured how fast each man walked when he joined the study. Then the researchers watched and waited for five years. In that time 266 men died. The average walking speed of the men joining the study was 0.88 metres per second (around 2 miles, or 3 kilometres, per hour), but of course some men walked a good bit faster than that. And remarkably *not a single man died* who could walk faster than 1.36 metres per second (3 miles, or 5 kilometres, per hour). As the researchers memorably put it, 'Faster speeds are protective against mortality because fast walkers can maintain a safe distance from the Grim Reaper.' They had worked out the walking speed of Death himself.

However, plenty of other research points to the benefits of being active beyond simply keeping us alive. All the worthy messages about smoking and drinking and taking statins and flossing our teeth don't do the 'compressed morbidity' trick; they help us live *longer* but don't necessarily make us live *healthier*. So far the only thing that has been shown consistently to increase life expectancy *and* allow those extra years to be spent in good health is getting off our bottoms.

Exercise! The very word makes many of us want to snuggle deeper into an armchair, yet it's worth having a brief thump on the exercise drum because it truly is one of the things that helps us stay well and independent towards the end of our lives. In fact, we don't have to do much to make a meaningful difference, because we're starting from such a low baseline. Human beings really are staggeringly idle, and lots of people just do not move for whole hours at a stretch.

Simply standing up from time to time would be a good start.

Snippets of information are gathering into an international voice that calls on us to get moving. In the UK my colleague Rob Andrews works in a team that has looked at the blood sugar levels of office workers after a meal. They've shown that sugar falls to safe levels in those who stand up for two minutes in every twenty, rather than remaining seated. Their sugar levels drop even further – a good thing – if they walk around a bit for those two minutes. It's not just sugar levels. From Brazil to New Zealand studies show that falls, and fear of falling, can be reduced by exercise in very old people, especially by activities that focus on muscle strength and balance. And, again in Australia, another study group called DYNOPTA (Dynamic Analyses to Optimize Ageing) are finding that the difference between being sedentary and moving about is a real reduction in years spent with disability in later life.

Reassuringly it's those who do the least exercise who benefit most from making a small change. And even more comfortingly increasing physical activity makes a difference even when we're already super old. Being active helps us to remain healthy and to keep our independence.

Returning to my graphs of 'life curve' (see pages 32 and 33), what's been happening for the last few decades has been a gradual extension of overall life expectancy to the right. But the curve hasn't kept up with the increase in life expectancy – it has shifted a little but not enough. So more people are spending extra time with disability down in that bottom right-hand corner of the graph – high age, low independence – where things get tricky.

In Newcastle, Professor Carol Jagger and her team have been looking at how we live longer. They've studied the life expectancy of people aged sixty-five and how it has changed. In 1991 women who were already sixty-five could expect to live about sixteen more years. Twenty years later, in 2011, similar women could instead expect about another twenty years – there was a 'bonus' of almost four years. For the sixty-five-year-old men the life expectancy bonus was even bigger, four and a half extra years. However, when the team looked at disability, measured by how well people could manage a variety of daily tasks like dressing and cooking, the results were not so good, especially for women. Of all the 'bonus' time the 2011 group of women could expect to live, only six months would be healthy – the other three extra years would be spent with some level of disability. In both men and women the overall proportion of life spent without disability had *reduced* over the two decades.

The Newcastle team are famously positive, and they looked more carefully at the data, dividing disability into mild and severe, and they found that most, though not all, of the extra 'disabled years' would be with mild rather than severe disability. They also sensibly looked at how people rate themselves, studying a measure of self-perceived health collected by the Office for National Statistics. More optimistically it turned out that, despite the increase in disability, the 2011 group rated their health better than the 1991 group. But we can't get away from the fact that people entering old age now are less fit than old people were twenty or thirty years ago. All the evidence from around the world, from Newcastle to Hong Kong, suggests that the picture is getting worse, and it's likely that our sedentary and greedy lifestyle is firmly to blame. To be fair this isn't really news: Cicero observed over 2,000 years ago that 'intemperate and indulgent youth will bring to old age a feeble and worn-out body'.

Here is the plan. This is not about Fitbits and Lycra. In fact, although it's great being super active, those at the top end of the scale don't gain much by increasing their activity yet further. The biggest benefits are to be won by persuading the rest of us to make the change from doing almost nothing to moving around a little bit more. In super-old age it's being able to move from sitting to standing up without someone helping that changes everything. Muir Gray, a distinguished public health physician, has written a cheerful book called *Sod Seventy!*, which includes lots of sensible and realistic suggestions about exercise. But the bottom line is it really doesn't matter what we do; we just need to do a bit more of it. Get moving. Then move a bit more. That's it.

However, successful old age is clearly not just about physical health. Some people seem to be good at being old. I met Diana a few times in clinic while we sorted out an attack of polymyalgia rheumatica.* She had been injured in a car accident in her early seventies and had used a wheelchair ever since. She was eighty-one, radiated contentment, and showed me pictures on her phone of her grandchildren, about whom she was relentlessly positive ('That one's Erin, she's such a keen little reader, and here is Jonno – I've never met a kinder young man.'). I admired how she kept in touch with them via Facebook and listened to their worries. 'I'm trying to be a good granny. I wasn't a very good mother,' Diana told me. I demurred. I couldn't imagine her being anything

---

* Polymyalgia is a poorly understood condition. No one knows why it happens, and some doctors don't believe it exists at all; they feel their colleagues are failing to find some other diagnosis that explains the symptoms. However, the classic picture is of a rapid onset over a few days of severe pain and stiffness in the muscles of the shoulders and thighs. It's worst first thing in the morning, and there's usually an association with other symptoms like loss of appetite and a sudden lowering of mood. Blood tests show a high level of inflammation, but there's no evidence of an infection, and the symptoms respond rapidly to steroids. The problem is, lots of things cause aches and pains and get a bit better with steroids, and older people often have slightly high levels of inflammation for other reasons, so polymyalgia is a diagnosis that's easy to get wrong. And making the wrong diagnosis is important because long-term treatment with steroids comes with loads of side effects, many of which can't be reversed.

but a model of maternal perfection, but she waved me down.

'No, honestly . . . I was so bound up in my marriage, and having a glamorous time, travelling and things, I just sent my children off to boarding school. And they told me they didn't like it, and I told them it was good for them . . . and I look back now and think whatever was I doing?'

Diana's words made me realize that different people often seem to be good at being different ages. The terrible toddler, the despair of his mother, may grow up to become an energetic, risk-embracing entrepreneur; the gloomy introspective teenager dressed in Goth clothes chooses to put herself through a process of hard-won insight and becomes a careful and empathetic teacher. Conversely school superstars can sag in midlife, dragged down by unrealized dreams. And some people seem to have a knack for being old. For many this may be a natural evolution: being disinclined to worry and having a ready sense of humour are ingrained traits that are likely to stand one in good stead when the going gets tough.

The good news is that it looks as if there is a natural and worldwide tendency for people to become happier as they age. Jonathan Rauch's book, *The Happiness Curve*, describes research from many countries indicating that human beings as a rule are reasonably happy in their twenties, become less happy in midlife, and cheer up again as they get older. The bottom of the happiness curve in the UK is around the age of forty-nine, so it's a nice book to give someone for a fiftieth birthday present. On average, Rauch suggests, everything's going to start feeling better once you've made the half-century. However, the research in Rauch's book seems to stop around the age of seventy-five, and it's not clear what happens after that. For some, illness will make happiness elusive; others seem to weather the grimmest of medical problems with a sunny smile. Many people hold a theory that character traits become more accentuated as we age — so the meticulously tidy person becomes obsessive, and the curmudgeonly fellow becomes aggressively reclusive, but that's not always true. Certainly dementia can change a personality utterly for good or bad (Martha described how her father, a stickler for rigid routines, became 'almost easy-going' as he became more forgetful), but more importantly we do each have some choice about how well we age. We can look after ourselves physically, but we can also make positive decisions about how we greet the world, which can make things better for ourselves and those we love.

I often ask my oldest patients what the secret has been of their long and healthy lives. There are recurrent themes. Don't worry. Be contented. Keep active. I'm shown crosswords, Sudokus and word searches, and am told of projects and passions. One of our standardized memory assessments includes a requirement for the patient to write a sentence. 'You can write anything you like,' I say as I hand over the pen. The sentences are scored boringly, for containing a verb and a noun and making sense, but provide insights into psychological well-being more revealing than retention of the rules of grammar. 'It's a lovely day' or 'I don't like tests', or 'I wish I was in the garden'. Derek took ages writing his sentence, and handed it over: 'I hope this won't take long, as I need to get back to my workshop in which I am recreating a fifteenth-century Italian painting using egg tempera.' There are hints of isolation or low mood, and, conversely, statements conveying intellectual and physical activity, interest, joy.

What are the other steps my patients have taken, that have helped them be happy as well as healthy in super-old age? This list may risk stating the obvious and many are definitely easier said than done, but here are some of the tips I've been given. Repeatedly I've been told: 'Take each day as it comes', 'Stop worrying'. Equally I'm advised to make good plans for the future: write a will, tidy my desk, make sure my family will know where to find my life insurance policy. Go on holiday. Do more, not less. Try not to be defeated by new technology – Cecil described how long it had taken him to get to grips with his iPhone, but now he was able to FaceTime his son's family in Los Angeles. 'Be willing to move house at the right moment,' said Anne, relieved to be closer to her daughter, but Charles told me, 'I'm prepared to fight to the end to stay in my own home', before dying a few weeks later, just yards from the room in which he had been born.

I've been told: 'Try to be easy to help', 'Accept what you can't do', 'Allow others to help you'. But I have been told this always by the spouse, the daughter, the would-be helper, while the unwilling recipient sets her jaw or has a glint in his eye, so perhaps the advice should be 'Accept that it may not be possible to help', which itself is a very hard thing to be told. 'Make peace with old enemies', Harry advised, 'Set things right.'

Perhaps the most useful advice came from Jack who shared his secret when I saw him in clinic following a couple of falls probably related to his horrible arthritis. He swayed into the consulting room, bent at the hips and grasping a stick in each lumpy hand. I could hear crunching from his knees as he sat down. Tweed jacket, Tattersall check shirt, cricket-club tie, pale blue lambs-wool V-neck. We went through things carefully – there was no suggestion of blackouts or funny turns – Jack's heart and lungs seemed in good order, his feet knobbly but reasonably functional, no medications. His son and daughter-in-law sat sturdily opposite him. Now ninety-six, Jack had been a farmer – like many locally he had kept mixed stock, with beef cattle and a small milking herd, some sheep and a few acres of hay and silage. He liked the cows best. We had a chat about his arthritis, and the pros and cons of joint replacements, but Jack wasn't keen, especially as all of his joints were in a shocking state, and it wasn't clear where an orthopaedic surgeon should start. I promised a visit from the therapy team to look into getting some extra bits and pieces at home – rails by the toilet, a seat in the shower, a neat bit of kit called a bed lever that slides under the mattress and produces a handle to hang on to while trying to get past the creaky start of the day. 'Apart from your joints, Jack, you are in amazing shape. What's the secret then?' Jack grinned, and glanced at his daughter-in-law, who twitched her chin and looked at the ceiling. Jack bent forward. 'I'll tell 'ee, Doctor Porlick.' He had lowered his voice, and I had to lean towards him. His eyes were china blue and he spoke very slowly. 'I never touched a drink . . . or a cigarette . . . or a woman . . . till I were ten.'

4. 'Good News!'

When someone develops a tight ache across the chest, worsened by exertion and perhaps associated with pain in the arm or jaw, they guess that they may have angina, and know that they would like to visit a cardiologist. Increasing pain in an arthritic hip prompts a trip to the GP and a request for referral to an orthopaedic surgeon. The diverse crowd in the waiting room of the sexual health clinic have chosen to go there; they know which specialist they need. But nobody asks to see a geriatrician. Patients arrive in our clinics already on the back foot, disturbed to have received a letter summoning them to an appointment in the department of geriatric medicine (or the department for medicine of old age, or for care of older people, or some other euphemistic expression that cuts no ice). It's often apparent that their GP hasn't quite come clean when suggesting the referral – our patient may have been offered 'a specialist review' or 'a thorough check-over'; no one said anything about 'geriatric'. It's not only those whom we see in clinic who take a dim view of being referred to our specialty – the patients who arrive desperately unwell on our acute wards look around at their companions in nearby beds and confide to their families that 'the staff are nice, but everyone else in here is *old*'. Our patients are often not at all sure what the geriatrician might be up to – perhaps we are going to break dire news, or are scheming to have them taken into care, or both. There's a wariness, and trust must be built. What is it that geriatricians do?

'Good news!' Mum announced.

I waited. This wouldn't necessarily be good news.

'We've booked a holiday in Costa Rica!'

Mum pointed to a brochure lying on top of the pile of paper that was threatening to slide into her cereal bowl. It had a glossy yellow cover with a vivid photograph of a green tree frog.

At the time my dear stepdad was only eighty-nine and in good shape. A couple of years previously, he and Mum had been to Uzbekistan, spotting birds and visiting mosques. Since then he had lost a little height and carried a slightly bewildered look on first waking from a post-lunch nap. But his pacemaker was checked regularly and he walked down to the shop each day to buy *The Times*. Perhaps a trip to Costa Rica would be fine, provided they took it easy.

'It's an adventure holiday!' Mum continued. 'We start with a beach bit, seeing the turtles, then stay a few nights in the cloud forest, and there are walking tours and rope bridges.'

'Oh. That sounds . . . exciting.'

I looked at the brochure. She'd turned down the

corner of the page showing the holiday she'd chosen and had circled some of the options. 'Dolphin watching' was highlighted, together with 'kayaking through the mangroves'. She had passed up on the zip wire and the waterfall rappelling.

Mum is younger than my stepdad by twelve years, but has had more than her share of medical problems. When she was in her early seventies a tumour grew deep behind her eyes, giving her double vision. The tumour was zapped by radiotherapy, but the radiation destroyed her pituitary, the tiny powerhouse of hormonal activity that nestles in the centre of the brain. Mum now needed daily doses of replacement hormones to regulate her metabolism, and steroids to keep her adrenalin at a life-sustaining level. The steroids had rendered her skin almost as thin and brittle as rice paper, and she had taken to wearing gloves when handling letters in order to avoid cuts. Additionally, several decades previously, her spine had set off on a mysterious but determined journey, simultaneously twisting to the right at its base, and to the left higher up, and tilting forward. One of my colleagues in the spinal surgical team had made a valiant attempt to constrain her wandering vertebrae using a framework of titanium posts, plates and screws, but over the years her bones had taken their own course again, warping the framework and pulling away from it, like the barky stem of an ancient rose forcing itself away from a trellis. Having been a tall woman, she was now no higher than my chest and was bent to such an angle that she had to lean her head towards her shoulder and tip herself sideways to gain eye contact. I glanced down again to check the flight details: check-in at Gatwick, 27 June, 0700.

'All sorted,' said Mum firmly, patting the brochure with a gloved hand. 'And they'll do us a special bird safari.'

In early July I bumped into Mum's endocrinologist Edmund in the corridor at work. A clever and meticulous doctor, he had looked after her hormone treatments for years, tweaking her doses to keep her pituitary replacement in order.

'How's your mother?' he asked.

I explained that she was away and outlined the itinerary. Edmund's eyebrows shot up above his gold-rimmed glasses.

'Costa Rica? Jeepers, Lucy, I'd have thought she'd be better off aiming for Costa Coffee.'

There's an odd thing that happens when people are talking about independence in the context of those who are becoming very old or frail. No one seems able to resist using the phrase 'fiercely independent', especially when they are talking about women. In fact, the smaller the old lady, the more likely she is to attract the label. It comes with a hint perhaps that she should be meeker, more willing to accept her ageing. Families and professionals worry about the well-being of our oldest people and their vulnerability. Edmund was not alone in his concern for my mum and stepfather, and their Central

American expedition had set the rest of the family a-jangle too.

Sometimes when those around the older person describe them as 'fiercely independent', they really mean 'selfishly independent' or 'stupidly independent'. As my friend Sally honestly remarked, despairing of her fragile father's habits of getting fish hooks in his fingers and lighting unruly bonfires in his garden, 'It's such a nuisance when he hurts himself.' But we also admire that independence, and we know it is what we would want for our own future.

The preservation of independence is undertaken mostly, of course, not by doctors but by people themselves just getting on with life. We don't need advice on how to grow old; it seems to come naturally. We walk the dog or sail single-handed round the world, stay up late to watch the Masters, attend mosque, church or synagogue, write furiously to the local paper, book ourselves on to bargain coach tours of the Cornish Riviera or the Norfolk Broads. Eighty is the new sixty, we are told, and it really is, as most of the twentieth-century gains in longevity are spent in good health, notwithstanding the tricky bit towards the end. As Libby Purves puts it, 'Sometimes on the Alps there are days when you can hardly throw a stick without hitting a retired headmistress on a mountain bike.' And it is said of Jeanne Calment, who lived to be 122, that on one of her many birthdays a young journalist impertinently asked, 'Madame, should I expect to be able to interview you again this time next year?', to which she replied, 'I don't see why not. You look in quite good health to me.'

However, for almost everyone, independence is inevitably threatened by ageing. The body's repair mechanisms that have sustained and protected us since infancy are not inexhaustible. If we must be fierce to defend our independence, we deserve allies.

The medical work to preserve independence is done to a large degree in primary care, by GPs and their teams, carefully shepherding the ageing body between safe boundaries – maintaining blood pressure within reasonable limits, spotting and treating reversible causes of decline. Gradually the list of long-term conditions may mount up, and although many GPs are accomplished in the care of people with complex problems, at some point it may become impossible to manage those problems within the standard ten-minute consultation. Or a new event or symptom hints at trouble that demands specialist knowledge, or access to diagnostic tests not available in primary care. A fall perhaps, or tremor, or weakness. Difficulty with memory, or with continence. Breathlessness, or loss of weight. A first appointment in a geriatric medicine clinic is long – half an hour at least, often forty-five minutes. Geriatricians are given time to tackle complexity. We have access too to a comprehensive list of colleagues: physios and occupational therapists, speech therapists, social workers, mental health nurses, dieticians and continence specialists, pharmacists and nurses with extraordinary knowledge of Parkinson's disease, heart failure, epilepsy. We have contact details for volunteers, who might visit, encourage, share sadness and laughter, support carers. Geriatric medicine is the ultimate team-based specialty.

Preserving independence is one thing; getting things back on track when they have been knocked sideways is another. Much of our work, and that of our junior doctors, is with the seriously sick, those admitted as an emergency, and here our role is often a sort of 'search and rescue' mission; quick decisions are needed, for our patient is grey and clammy, and the wolves of sepsis or multiple organ failure are snapping at their heels. And after the rescue mission may come a longer, more complicated process, which is about the restoration of independence.

Kathleen Graham had arrived at the community hospital; we'd been awaiting her for days. She'd broken her hip while visiting a friend on the other side of the country, and there'd been a row about who should pay for the ambulance transfer back here, closer to home.

I glanced in as I passed her room. She was still asleep, propped up in the bed, her chin on her chest. She was wearing the standard pink NHS nightie, one size fits nobody. Her suitcase sat by the locker, not yet unpacked – yesterday's journey had been long.

I slung my bag under the nurses' desk and flicked through the summary sent by the hospital 200 miles away. Kathleen had spent almost ten weeks there.

Fall, Left #NOF, DHS.

She had had a fractured neck of femur, the standard broken hip, patched together with a dynamic hip screw.

CAP, AKI: these are problems that commonly befall someone who is properly old and has broken a major bone. Kathleen had community acquired pneumonia when she was admitted – perhaps that was what had caused her to fall – and acute kidney injury; her kidneys' function had been hit, probably by a combination of blood loss and infection, and maybe some of her drugs. I read on.

Pneumonia treated, AKI resolved. Good.

UTI, delirium. Bad. She had developed a urine infection and had become confused.

Fall on ward, R tibial plateau fracture, NWB 12/52.

I winced. Poor Mrs Graham. These are words that speak of prolonged pain and unhappiness. The tibial plateau makes up the supporting surface of the knee joint; it takes all our weight when we stand and is hard to fix. Usually, as in Kathleen's case, the treatment is simply rest, which means keeping all pressure off the joint; she is to be *NWB*, non weight-bearing, for twelve weeks. Someone in better health might hop around, using crutches, but with her hip fracture on the other side that would be a challenge for Kathleen. I quickly scanned her background history: *I*: independent. *Lives alone, still drives.*

It can be tricky to work out what the chances of recovery are for a properly old person who has had a major illness or injury. Many sail through an event like a hip fracture, avoid complications through a combination of good care and good luck, and are back home within a few days, gathering their confidence once more. Others have a bumpier ride. For some the fracture is the end point of a downhill journey that has been evolving over several years. They are already at the gossamer-thread stage of life, and that thread is broken as surely as the hip bone itself – the frailest may die in hospital. For others, those with pre-existing problems, the fracture represents a major but not insuperable challenge; they need prolonged rehabilitation and attention to detail from a careful team, and slowly, steadily they get better. And then there are people like Kathleen Graham, caught up in a miserable game of snakes and ladders, and it's not clear whether they're going to be the winner.

Later, Liv the staff nurse and I reached Mrs Graham on our ward round. She was awake now, and someone had unpacked her suitcase, but her head was still hanging forward and she looked exhausted. I hunkered down by her bed, my elbow brushing against the catheter bag clipped to the bed frame. I introduced myself and Liv and touched Kathleen's hand.

'I'm really sorry you've been through the mangle. You must have had a rotten time.'

She raised her head slowly. She had grey-green eyes rimed with sleepy dust, and sparse lashes beneath high-arched brows. There were deep runnels from her nose to the sides of her mouth, and sore red creases ran down from the corner of her lips on each side. Her eyes closed and she shook her head just once. She whispered, 'I can't do this.'

Dr Mary Tinetti is Chief of Geriatrics at Yale School of Medicine. From her earliest career she studied the factors that contribute to falling in old people, based on work done mainly in the UK by the pioneers of geriatric medicine. In 1994 Tinetti led a team that demonstrated that the risk of having a fall could be reduced by sensible actions, such as stopping certain medications and doing exercises to improve strength. Their research was published in the *New England Journal of Medicine*, a prestigious journal with a reputation for serious science; other papers in that week's edition included work on DNA analysis in a rare genetic condition and a study comparing the effectiveness of various steroids in the treatment of Crohn's disease. Tinetti's paper was important, firstly because it showed conclusively that falls, previously considered an inevitable part of ageing, are in part preventable. She and her team also demonstrated that research about ageing didn't have to be based on the structural features of the senescent chromosome (how our genetic material alters with age) or pharmacokinetic changes in ageing kidneys (how they handle drugs), important though these are. They showed that it was possible to study, in a rigorous way, the effect of simple practical changes in the lives of real people.

Later in her career, Tinetti, now a professor of

medicine with multiple awards to her name, was asked to describe what geriatricians do and found herself at a loss. How could she succinctly describe our work? Eventually Tinetti came up with five Ms. She started at the top. Her first M is 'Mind', which encompasses mentation (thinking) as well as the three nasty Ds geriatricians must tackle: dementia, delirium and depression. Next comes 'Mobility': the importance of maintaining our ability to move around, and what we can do to help our patients to remain upright. Tinetti's third 'M' is 'Medication': geriatricians recognize that drugs have downsides, and that very old or frail people may have both most to gain and most to lose from what their doctors prescribe. Fourth, she identified 'Multicomplexity'. In this lumpy word she captures the need to be a good physician with the knowledge and patience to reach the right diagnosis (usually several diagnoses for our patients), but also the common sense to put those diagnoses into context for each individual. Tinetti uses 'multicomplexity' rather than the more common 'multimorbidity' to acknowledge what she calls the 'bio-psycho-social' complexity of the human being. Diagnostic accuracy is an essential component of good care, but it's no good just trying to fix the diseases without considering the patient's relationship with family and friends, and how they live their lives.

Back in the side room, I could hear Liv at the basin behind me; without looking I knew that she was washing Kathleen's glasses. I explained to Kathleen that I was going to examine her, not for too long, so that we could make a plan. I checked that she knew where she was; she couldn't quite recall the name of the little hospital we were in, but she knew she was back in her own county, and could tell me her date of birth and her age (eighty-eight) and the current year. I promised not to ask her any more daft questions and I felt her pulse, lifting her hand; her fingernails were ragged and ridged, and there was something grubby under them. When I asked her to, Kathleen opened her mouth, but not wide. I could see the cracks at the side of her lips – they hurt – and her tongue was smooth and shiny. Liv leaned over my shoulder to shine her pen torch into Kathleen's mouth; there were white patches dotted over the back of her throat. I turned Kathleen's head away, so that I could look at the veins of her neck – they're like a pressure gauge for the heart, pulsing faintly just above her collarbone. There was a gold chain and a locket and a small round medallion with an image of St Christopher carrying the baby Jesus. I slid my hand through the V of the pink nightie, and under her left breast (silky, flat), and could feel her heartbeat pressing hard, insistently, under my fingertips. My stethoscope had become tangled with the lanyard of the name badge round my neck, and while I was sorting it out Kathleen's head fell forward again. I put the stethoscope to her chest and listened to the blow of a murmur, like a stiff brush on a stone floor. I moved the stethoscope to the side of her neck and it was there too, the sound of an aortic valve that had narrowed, the flow of blood from her heart noisy as it rushed through the stenosis. Kathleen's eyes were closed – was she asleep, or simply staying out of this process?

Liv and I moved Kathleen's nightie so we could see her abdomen – the skin was folded and criss-crossed with tiny lines. There was a sprinkling of bright red dots, each a couple of millimetres across. They're Campbell de Morgan spots, harmless, which come with age ('signs of wisdom', a chest physician in east London, on the point of retirement himself, had taught me). Her tummy was soft beneath my hand, but her forehead ruffled.

'When did you last have a good bowel movement?' I asked.

She looked at me. 'I don't know . . . a few days?'

'I mean a proper turn-out?'

She shook her head. Liv moved the sheet, and we looked at Kathleen's legs; the left hip fracture wound had healed perfectly – there was a pink line only a couple of inches long with faint dots either side where the staples had punctured her skin. But her right leg was caged from thigh to ankle, gripped by a brace of thick neoprene and Velcro with steel brackets either side of her knee. In the gaps between the fabric I could see grey-green old bruises over the broken joint. The lower end of the brace had sunk into the puffy skin just above Kathleen's ankle – I touched it and felt the yielding marshmallow of oedema. Her left leg was the same: the bones of her ankle were indistinct under a cushion of fluid, and my fingers left dimples in the skin at the back of her calf.

I looked up at Kathleen's face, still dropping to her chest. 'Mrs Graham, we're going to gently, gently lift your legs.'

Liv and I lifted each leg in turn, bending our heads and squinting sideways to see dark mulberry circles under each heel. The weight of Kathleen's legs, heavy on the air mattress, was funnelled to a point of pressure high enough to interrupt blood supply and damage the fragile tissue over the heel bones. On the left her skin had already broken – there was a hole and a white ring of dead skin and an ooze of clear yellow fluid. We straightened up, and Liv lifted the brake under the bed with her foot.

'Kathleen, we've nearly finished. We're going to pop you a bit flatter and roll you over a little so I can have a listen to your chest and we can check that your bottom's not sore.'

Kathleen raised a thumb in assent, and we moved the bed away from the wall and lowered its head and rolled her sideways. I listened to the shush of her breath sounds between pale ribs, and we checked the skin of her bottom, rosy pink and undamaged, and then we rearranged the pillows behind her shoulders into an inverted V and rolled her back and propped her up, and she closed her eyes again while Liv and I picked up the charts of her observations and drugs.

I talked to Kathleen as we worked. 'I'm going stop a

couple of your tablets, because your blood pressure's on the low side now. And I'd like you to have the paracetamol regularly so you don't have to have to wait to be in pain before you get it – we can do it as a syrup if you can't manage the tablets – and I've written up some stronger stuff if you need it. But the stronger painkillers are all very binding and you'll need a laxative, because even if you're not eating, your insides still need to get moving. We're going to give you a bit of rocket fuel to sort those bowels out.'

I was watching Kathleen's face and there was a tiny twitch of the side of her lips. I wrote up the laxatives, together with some treatments for the thrush in her mouth, a common legacy of antibiotics, and I put in a request for some blood tests – levels of vitamins, and ferritin to check her iron supplies. Liv brought in a pair of foam boots, their heels cut away to take the pressure off Kathleen's sore points.

I crouched down again beside Kathleen and touched her hand. She pushed her eyes open one more time. 'You really have been through it. But . . . Liv and I think you can get better.'

Her head lolled. For a moment I looked past Kathleen, out to the garden where John, one of the occupational therapists, had hung bird feeders. There was a blue tit upside down on some nuts.

'Mrs Graham, Kathleen, please may I ask, what is the thing you're most worried about right now?'

Her gaze shifted over my shoulder, and I turned to

see the bedside table. There was a photograph, black and white in a silver frame. A man in a dinghy, one hand on the rudder, the other gripping the rail of the little boat. His hair was waving in the wind and he had a pipe clenched between his teeth. His eyes were alight with excitement and joy.

Kathleen whispered, 'I just want to go home.'

Dr Tinetti's final M is 'what Matters Most'. It's easy to forget what matters most in this world of high-tech medicine, of complex treatment options, of urgency and treatment algorithms, sepsis bundles and door-to-needle times. Atul Gawande recognizes the importance of 'what matters most' too, in his beautiful and sympathetic book *Being Mortal*, with its subtitle *Medicine and What Matters in the End*. Gawande explains through a series of case studies, including that of his own father, how often medical decisions are not clear cut; he describes how choice is present more often than we might think, and he explains how the right path might be chosen only when we are able to be honest about our hopes, fears and goals. The US Institute for Healthcare Improvement now encourages medical teams to find out not 'What is the matter with you?' but rather 'What matters to you?'

Coming to a correct diagnosis is important, and a patient's advanced age is no excuse for sloppy assessment; geriatricians sigh wearily at the 'go-to' diagnosis of urinary tract infection, beloved by time-pressured

medics but often wrong. Much unhappiness, pain and
wasted resources may result from failure to find out
exactly what the matter is with the patient. But as to
what matters *to* our patient, for that there's no fancy
scan. Working out what matters most isn't just a thing
with words, simply hearing the answer to a question. It
may be hidden: in the movement of a very old lady's
right hand over her left, as she feels for her wedding
ring; or in the look that passes between a daughter and
her father when she opens a *tadka dal* brought from
home; or in the glitter shed onto a bedside table by a
great-grandchild's get-well card. What matters most
might be hinted at: in a man's tired eyes sliding sideways
when the possibility of chemotherapy is mentioned, or
in the quick glance my patient throws towards her handbag when I ask her how often she finds she needs to take
a tablet to calm her nerves.

The nurses and healthcare assistants often work it out
earlier than me – they notice the fear expressed without
words during a long night, of being left alone; the hope
confided while sheets are being changed of being well
enough to attend a best friend's ninetieth birthday
party. The therapists who work in geriatric teams also
understand the importance of what matters most. They
know that if what *they* think matters, and what *their patient*
thinks matters, are two different things, their efforts
will be fruitless. They might frame the conversation
around 'goal setting' – today we agree that you will aim
to sit on the edge of the bed for five minutes. Tomorrow

you might sit in the chair. Next week, practise some stairs, make a cup of tea. The most perceptive therapists develop a talent for detecting when their goals and those of their patient are subtly diverging, and they explore or explain, cajole or compromise, to get things back on track.

There's a subsidiary meaning to Tinetti's 'what matters most'. The goals of our patient are key, but geriatricians also have to prioritize our interventions from an often long list of problems. Balance is needed between our instinct towards diagnostic purism, and a recognition that our patient may not benefit from the investigations and treatments we propose. There is a sensible saying that the science of medicine lies in knowing what to do, while the art may lie in knowing when not to do it. Some things do not need fixing.

For many years I used to give the medical students a lift to the community hospital in order that they could see something of rehabilitation in action. I'd sweep copies of the *BMJ* from the passenger seat and gather up the children's felt-tips, and the student would cautiously get in, and halfway through the fifteen-minute journey they would almost always draw my attention to a crack in the windscreen, a star in the glass quite low down.

'Did you know there's a crack there, Doctor P?' the student would offer. 'You could get that repaired.'

And each time, I would explain that the crack had been there for years, and that because it didn't interfere with the view of the road, the car was still safe and still passed its MOT.

On week two of her long, slow campaign for recovery, one of the students met Kathleen. He listened to her heart murmur, and he and I talked about aortic stenosis, and its association with blackouts and the risk of sudden death. We discussed what might be done about it – an echocardiogram back in the big hospital to assess its severity, followed by a decision: open surgery versus the newer, less invasive transcatheter aortic valve implant-ation, both performed in the regional cardiothoracic centre sixty miles down the road. Then we talked with Kathleen again, and the student looked at her leg in its neoprene and steel cage, and realized that the level of protein in her blood was still miles below its normal level, and then Kathleen sneezed, and she reached for a tissue and the student noticed that she did not have the strength even to pull a tissue out of its box. So the plan must recede for a scan to assess that heart murmur. The murmur might matter, but not right now, not most.

It would take a horrible arrogance to suggest that I know everything that matters to my patient. I'm aware that our relationship is necessarily both superficial and transient, yet may have profound consequences. One of the joys of geriatric medicine is gathering the infor-mation to do the job properly. A dense historical biography, half read, or a prayer slip tucked beneath a vase of flowers; a piece of knitting; a phrase, a glance – of course these

are not observations on which to base important decisions, but they are clues left on the path. They're not
things to be judged, but they might start conversations,
or at least allow me a glimpse into hopes and fears. I'll
never really know what matters most, but must try to
have some understanding.

The next week, Kathleen was delirious, laid low by a
bout of norovirus that had torn through the ward. She'd
become dehydrated and was having some intravenous
fluid, but she looked terrible, and I wasn't sure she was
going to recover. Then I was away on holiday for a fort-
night and returned one Tuesday with the medical student
to the community hospital, glancing into rooms as we
walked to the nurses' station. Kathleen was reading, her
caged leg stretched out on a footstool, her table a clutter
of coffee cup, bourbon biscuits, parish magazine. Behind
her on the windowsill something small and bright
moved – a little plastic figurine, a curvaceous girl with
wavy black hair, a tiny waist, generous bosom and red
polka-dot bikini. A miniature solar panel at her base supplied power, and she wriggled her hips from side to side.

The student and I talked with Kathleen. She was
wearing a sweatshirt with a floral appliqué dog on it, and
an enormous gutter frame stood in the corner of the
room; it had wide padded arms so that Kathleen could
support herself when she practised standing on her left
leg for a few seconds at a time. The thrush in her mouth
had gone, as had the catheter, and her bowels had finally
achieved equilibrium, but she still had no appetite and

very little strength, and it would be many weeks yet until she'd be allowed to put weight through the right leg.

'You look a bit better,' I said, and she looked at me gloomily.

'I feel eurgh. I hate the hoist and everything tastes awful.'

'Would a tiny drop of sherry help?' I asked, and the student looked surprised, but Kathleen shrugged, and said, 'Worth a try,' so I wrote up a very small dose of sherry, telling Kathleen, 'It's only twenty mils, that's four teaspoons' worth, once a day, "as required", to boost your appetite.'

(There's always a bit of debate with pharmacy about whether I'm allowed to do this, but if I don't, I know that some of the nurses will fear she's not allowed to have it, even if her family bring it in, so I write it up and we muddle along.)

Liv came past us and looked at the chart, and said please would I also prescribe big doses of grit and determination, and the student looked at Kathleen and said he thought Mrs Graham had got those already, and Kathleen looked up at the student and winked, and she gave him a smile that I hope he'll remember for the rest of his career.

*

You can read Professor Tinetti's 1994 paper here:
https://www.nejm.org/doi/full/10.1056/NEJM199409
293311301

75

5. Four Things About Falls

I ask the three medical students to stand up, so they put down their folders and notebooks, and they stand in the messy office I share with Charlie, with its box files full of educational guidance, teaching assessment proformas and exam schedules. Information leaflets for Charlie's patients with Parkinson's disease flow from drawers, and our desks are piled with notes and letters and Post-its and sheets of photos of this year's cohort of trainee doctors.

The students think about what is keeping them upright; we observe that it took several million years of evolution for mankind's predecessors to stand on two feet, and that it's easy to wobble. They realize that they aren't standing stock still: all the time their muscles are twitching and adjusting to tiny changes in position, constantly pulling each body back to the vertical without conscious thought. The students remember their anatomy and physiology lessons, and tell me about the signals their brains are receiving – messages from tiny position detectors, proprioceptors, in their feet and around their knees and in the multiple small joints of their spines; messages from the delicate balancing mechanism of the inner ear; visual messages. I ask them to shut their eyes and they become unsteady and have to concentrate harder to stand still. The students notice next that in order to have perfect balance all the paths must be intact along which the messages from eyes, ears and feet are sent to the brain – paths along nerves and up the spinal cord. The brain must be working too, gathering all that information and interpreting it, then sending messages back, along intact pathways once more, to make the muscles move. The students can see that the muscles must be strong, and the load-bearing joints must be reliable. And the muscles, nerves and brain need a good supply of energy; for that the heart must be working properly, generating enough pressure to send blood through functioning arteries – arteries that themselves constrict and relax, continuously, imperceptibly, to keep the flow of blood perfect.

Now the students can see why they're going to have several lessons about falls, and why, when they become a doctor, their assessment of an older person who has fallen will be a more complicated matter than checking for bruises and breaks. What should my patients, and those who love and worry about them, also know about falls? What should they do or expect to be done?

Ellen is put out. She is sitting next to a bed in our acute medical unit, and tells me, 'I fell over in the garden, and now there's been a lot of brouhaha. And I heard the physio talking to that nurse; he said I'd had a fall, but I didn't "have a fall", I just fell over. Saying I had a fall makes me sound old.'

I glance at Ellen's date of birth. She's ninety-two.

Her left forearm is encased in a plaster cast; she broke her wrist when she fell, and the Emergency Department doctor has written 'FOOSH' in her notes, meaning Fall Onto OutStretched Hand. The doctor was clearly in a hurry, as ED doctors naturally must be; he has scribbled 'mechanical fall' and drawn a little outline of a heart and lungs and written 'clear'. Ellen is keen to get home, and I'm equally keen that she should go home. The physio has checked her over, and Ellen was able to leap in and out of bed, and she has been up the stairs, overtaking some poor middle-aged fellow as he climbed gingerly towards the cardiology lab. Jodie the OT has seen Ellen too. Put simply, physiotherapists find out and improve the movements you can make; occupational therapists, OTs, work on function – what you can actually do with the movement you have. Ellen proved herself nippy at getting in and out of her clothes despite the plaster cast, and Jodie has recorded that she 'cooks from scratch', noting with respect that for Ellen this means not only washing the leeks and potatoes for her soup but growing them too.

But I don't want to let Ellen go just yet. There are more questions to ask.

Jaz, one of the junior doctors, met Ellen late last night, after she'd been sent up from ED, and has presented her case to me.

'I'm not sure why she fell,' Jaz has told me, looking slightly grey in her navy night scrubs. Jaz needs to get home for a restless daytime sleep before her next shift, but she's done a thorough job with Ellen. 'She doesn't actually remember exactly what happened. She says she was in the garden, and then she was on the ground. I couldn't find anything much on examination and she's got perfect bloods.'

Jaz shows me the screen – all Ellen's blood results are blue, normal, which would be unusual in a thirty-year-old (there's almost always one result lying irrelevantly just outside the normal range) and is impressive at ninety-two. Jaz goes on, 'Her obs and ECG are fine. I've asked for lying and standing blood pressures.'

Jaz and I go to see Ellen together, and she repeats her story. Ellen wants to tell me about what happened after the fall: the shock of finding herself on the hard path; the knowledge, immediate and painful, that she'd broken her arm; the long wait for help; the neighbour passing with her baby in the pushchair. I need to listen, and to acknowledge how shaken Ellen is, despite her resolute stoicism, but what I really want to know is what happened *before* the fall, not after it. What's her walking usually like? Was she unwell in any way? Was there any warning?

'I must have tripped,' says Ellen, but she hadn't tripped.

'Ellen, do you remember the actual moment of hitting the ground?'

She looks at Jaz. 'Yes . . . well, no. Not the moment. I was on the ground.'

'Do you think you might have had a little blackout, just for a few seconds?'

'I might have,' she concedes.

'Has anything like that happened in the past?'

Ellen tells us about a fall a few weeks ago, in her lounge that time ('I just went down, but it was on the carpet'), and as she speaks her hand moves to touch a mark on her cheekbone; there's a pink scar, a left-handed tick, on her tanned face.

'Ow, that must have been sore. Did you see anyone, a doctor, after that fall?'

Ellen frowns. 'I don't like to make a fuss.'

One of the defining challenges for all of us as we get older is working out what we should expect of our bodies. Is this ache normal? Does everyone get up in the night for a pee? Is it OK to find I've put the orange juice in the oven? What is inevitable? What is reversible? Should I say 'Ah, well, these things happen?' Or should I make a fuss?

Many things that happen with ageing seem to be common; we know other people with those problems – uncles and in-laws and friends at the club, so we know 'these things happen', and are not surprised when they happen to us too. However, many of the difficulties that come with age are common but are not inevitable; they are not *normal*. So dementia is a common problem, but it is not a normal part of ageing. Problems with continence are common; they are not normal. Weight loss, ankle swelling, depression: all are common, but not normal.

Falling is common, but it is not normal.

Falls have causes, and causes can be identified, and we may be able, together, to do something about them.

In 1999 Jacqueline Close, then still a trainee doctor in geriatric medicine, did a trial to investigate how the risk could be reduced of falling again after a fall. She was working at King's College Hospital in south London, and looked at patients over the age of sixty-five who had come to the Emergency Department following a fall. The patients were divided randomly into two equally sized groups: one group got the intervention; the control group received 'usual care'.

Twelve months later, some patients had been lost to follow-up, but most had contributed to Jacqui's data. The total reported number of falls was 183 in the intervention group compared with 510 in the control group. The risk of having one further fall was dramatically reduced in the intervention group, and there was an even greater drop in their risk of recurrent falls. In addition, the odds of admission to hospital were lower in the intervention group, while the control group became significantly worse at carrying out everyday tasks.

What was it, this intervention that Dr, now Professor, Close and her colleagues had performed? Jacqui herself saw each of the patients assigned to the intervention

group, 152 of them, in her clinic, and quizzed them carefully about what had happened when they fell. She
examined them and measured their blood pressure
while they were lying down, and again after they stood
up, and she made them stand on one leg, and checked
their vision with an optician's chart. She asked about
medications and mood, and did a short test of cognition. Jacqui's colleague Margaret Ellis, an occupational
therapist, visited each of the intervention patients at
home, looking for risks that could be reduced, or adaptations that might be helpful, and recording what things
the patients could still do for themselves. Jacqui and
Margaret made suggestions. Medicines were stopped or
changed for some; others were referred for a pacemaker. Many were advised to visit an optician. Loose
rugs were removed or tacked down; sloppy slippers
went in the bin; handrails were installed. Almost everyone was offered some sort of intervention. The control
group received usual care: they were seen by the emergency team, patched up and either admitted or sent
home.

The trial was highly significant. The strength of a
trial's result, how much notice we should take of its
claims, is often measured by a 'p value', the lower the
better. In Jacqui's trial, the 'p value' for the reduction in
falls was 0.0002, meaning that there was only a 1 in 5,000
chance that this result could have come about by luck
alone. The findings were impressive, and, like Tinetti's
work five years previously, Jacqui Close's trial appeared

in a prestigious journal, this time *The Lancet*. Like Mary Tinetti, Jacqui became a professor of medicine. She moved to Sydney, where her department produces top-grade research on falls and their relation to dizziness, dementia, injuries and exercise – Jacqui's focus is on *function*; her team's research is centred on how to help older people maintain independence and joy. The care of those who have fallen demands a lively attention to diagnosis, together with an observant and imaginative response to practical reality: it's a team effort to study for each of us how our feet are planted on the ground, what is needed to keep us upright, and where we want each step to take us.

Back in the acute medical unit, Jaz and I talk with Ellen, and explain that it sounds as if her falls may have been due to blackouts, 'transient loss of consciousness'. She doesn't need to stay in hospital, but we need to do a little more work to find out why they're happening; Ellen's heart may be running much too fast or much too slow, just for a few moments, long enough to stop her heart from sending enough blood to her brain. By the time she lands on the floor the heart rhythm will have come back to normal – there'll be nothing to see on her ECG after the fall. Or it may be that her blood pressure is dropping unexpectedly; I explain to Ellen that this is a common problem as we age. The bouncy blood vessels of our youth have walls a bit like brand-new knicker elastic, and they squeeze when we stand to keep blood moving up to our brain. Blood vessels become stiff when we get older, and our blood pressure can be quite normal, or even high, when we're sitting, but may plummet when we get out of a chair or bed.

Ellen and I agree a plan. Later, I'll show the daytime trainee how to do a carotid sinus massage, a five-second rub of Ellen's neck that imitates a rise in blood pressure, triggering messages to the heart telling it to calm down, slow down: if her heart is prone to going too slowly, this trick may well provoke it to do just that. We'll have an ECG running and may be able to record her heart doing what it did when she fell. If the carotid massage doesn't show anything, Ellen will go home with a heart monitor on for a few days. She can take it off for her bath, but the rest of the time it'll stay there, silently watching. My guess is that we'll catch Ellen's heart on a go-slow, or even stopping completely for a few seconds; the cardiologists will be happy to fix that with a pacemaker. I hope Ellen may well be like some of the patients in Professor Close's trial, whose risk of falling was dramatically reduced by an intervention.

The most important thing Jacqui Close did in her study was to ask the geriatricians' favourite question, which is 'Why?' Simply asking 'Why?' is our most useful tool in tackling the conundrum of deciding whether 'this is common' or 'this is normal'. Why is this mild-mannered man driving his wife to distraction with his violent dreams of which he has no recollection? Why does this elegant woman have humiliating episodes of incontinence? And why exactly did this person fall and hurt themselves badly enough to have to come to hospital? Only after we've thought properly about why a fall occurred, can we move on to doing something about it.

So, dear Ellen, make a fuss. 'Fall' is a description, not a *diagnosis*, and you deserve a diagnosis.

Frustratingly, twenty years after Jacqui's trial, and despite a wealth of further studies showing what a difference can be made by a good assessment and attention to detail, people who come to ED after a fall are not guaranteed the service provided by Jacqui Close and Margaret Ellis. In some hospitals assessment for those who have fallen is slick and comprehensive, but in many it is not, and problems more complicated than loss of consciousness may go untackled. We often let people down (literally indeed) when we recognize that the fall may have been due to a combination of factors but fail to do enough about them. 'Mechanical fall' is often written, a shorthand label meaning 'it wasn't a blackout or a heart attack, a stroke or an infection; I think it was a trip'. The problem here is that the label suggests that nothing more needs to be done; that a trip in old age is normal as well as common.

Wilf is eighty-four and is a musician; he played the trumpet in cruise-ship bands. He's been picked up by the ambulance crew after spending a night on the floor. He told the crew he'd tripped on a rug. He is a big man and has diabetes and heart failure. I hear about what happened to Wilf from Dan, one of the trainees. We've been on call together a few times, and Dan teases me as we stand in the cramped doctors' office filled with the dusty air exhaled by computer hard drives.

'You're not going to want "mechanical fall", Doctor P; please can I write "multifactorial fall" instead?'

'Only if you can tell me fifteen factors and what you are going to do about them.'

Dan runs through things confidently. Wilf has diabetes, so will be prone to high or, worse, low sugars, which may make him confused and wobbly. The diabetes is likely to have affected his vision, through the development of cataracts or retinal damage, and diabetes also comes with neuropathy, damage to nerves; Wilf may not be able to feel his feet well, and the nerve damage will also affect his blood pressure control as nerves carry messages to blood vessels, telling them whether to constrict or relax, so his blood pressure may be fine when he's sitting, but may well drop when he stands. Some of his heart failure treatments may aggravate that. I'm listening to Dan and keep count. He has listed seven factors so far, some of which we can address. Dan continues. Wilf's heart failure is making his feet swollen, which will also interfere with sensation, that's eight. And his legs are big and heavy with fluid, oedema, and will be hard for him to move, nine, and his lungs are water-logged too, so the delivery of oxygen to his muscles and brain will be poor, ten. Dan picks up Wilf's drug list. As well as the heart failure drugs that push his blood pressure downwards, he's on an antidepressant, citalopram, and all antidepressants can aggravate postural drops in blood pressure, eleven. I have run out of fingers as Dan goes on. Wilf takes codeine for his arthritis; it may be making him confused, and Dan knows that walking is a very cognitive activity. Staying upright takes lots of brainpower, even when we're not consciously thinking about it, and anything that messes with our brain enough to make us confused also makes us more likely to fall. That's twelve. Wilf's taking gabapentin for diabetic neuropathic pain; in common with its sister drug, pregabalin, one of its most common side effects is ataxia, poor balance, thirteen.

Dan is doing well. He shows me Wilf's ECG – it's not great, and his heart disease may be provoking rhythm changes: too fast, too slow. Fourteen, fifteen. We look at Wilf's blood results: his essential water tablets, diuretics, have caused his kidneys to lose potassium, and low potassium levels make muscles weak, sixteen.

We haven't even touched yet upon Wilf's knees, his leaky bladder, his levels of hormones, vitamins, minerals; his cottage with its multiple small steps between kitchen, toilet and sitting room, his steep stairs; his diet of mainly custard creams and his slightly unexpected fondness for Tia Maria, which we discover only when his niece visits.

When Dan and I meet Wilf he's despondent. This has not been his first fall, and he looks down at the spreading violaceous bruise on his arm, then he gives a little wiggle in his chair, and smiles at Dan, and says, 'One of those things.'

But, Wilf, this fall is not 'one of those things'. It's 'lots of things', and we can make some of them better. We can change your medicines, improve your leg swelling, get your blood ingredients sorted; we can stop your sugar levels dropping out, and tweak things so your blood pressure is less likely to get too low; we can work on your strength and balance; we can think about what specs you are wearing, and we can take you home, where the therapists will look at what you can do, will move that mat, put in rails, raise the toilet seat, give you a stool to perch on at the sink.

Wilf, you might well fall again, whatever we do, and I don't know which of these changes, if any, is going to make a difference, but I know that if we respond, are active in looking for and solving problems, you will be less likely to fall again. You deserve detailed assessment and action.

The situation is even starker for those who have had a hip fracture, when the difference between action and inaction can be counted in deaths. The National Hip Fracture Database was set up by the Royal College of Physicians and encourages orthopaedic teams to work together with geriatricians to improve care. And it works. The NHFD team publish data describing the care of almost every hip fracture patient, every year, in every hospital in England, Wales and Northern Ireland (Scotland does its own thing) and have worked with those providing the money, clinical commissioning groups, to encourage hospitals to invest in better services. Hospitals get extra cash if they fulfil certain criteria, such as ensuring that patients get their fracture-fixing operation promptly, providing weekend physio and looking out for new or worsening confusion. Simple things, like getting someone out of bed quickly after their operation (often to the alarm of their family), and providing protein-boosting supplements, translate into real benefits: a shorter hospital stay, a better chance of getting home. To earn the bonus payments, hospitals must show that each patient is seen by an orthogeriatrician, a doctor who specializes in the care of older people who have broken bones. Orthogeriatricians attend to medical complexities and think about the cause of the fall, and plan bone-strengthening strategies to reduce the risk of another fracture.

Internationally there's recognition that it's worth getting this complicated care right: inspired by the National Hip Fracture Database team's results, there's now a Global Fragility Fracture Network, which links passionate activists in India, China, Malaysia, Brazil – all determined to improve outcomes. Hospitals in Australia and New Zealand have replicated the NHFD work, and in 2017 they found that in the best-performing hospital almost everyone who came in from their own home with a hip fracture had returned to their own home within 120 days. In the worst only just over half had made it home. In the UK, 3% of those treated in the best hospital had died within thirty days; in the hospitals that performed worst one in ten had died.

The NHFD's carrot and stick approach has dragged standards up, but they are not met in every hospital in the UK, and there's been a recent wobble in the previously steady line of improvement; the average wait for surgery had become a few painful hours longer in 2017 and 2018 compared with 2015, and the authors of the report express their concern that this 'may be indicative of rising pressure on theatre capacity'. But they also note that teams report inefficiencies in their own use of operating theatre time, with 'lists routinely starting late and the avoidable cancellation of individual cases'. Case studies are used to show how the best hospitals achieve their results, and the NHFD authors don't let poorly performing teams off the hook easily. In his foreword to the 2018 report the then president of the British Orthopaedic Association, Ananda Nanu, called for 'sober analysis of the reasons for variation in units and an honest appraisal of shortcomings in resources, personnel and attitudes'.

Those who have fallen deserve a proper diagnosis, and action from professionals, and patients and their families can help call us to account. It's not about complaining or making life miserable for individual staff; it's about having realistic expectations of what can be done. It's reasonable for a patient to ask why did I fall, and is there anything that can be done about it, and am I getting the care that has been shown to make a difference?

We can also do much to help ourselves. I visited Bert in his second-floor flat years ago. He had refused to come to clinic, because he looked after his wife Queenie, who had dementia, and he would not leave her side. There were concerns about his unsteadiness, a question as to whether he might have Parkinson's disease. I couldn't see how he'd escaped a fall so far. I let myself into the flat using the key code his GP had supplied, and despite my protests Bert stood up to shake my hand. He had a tremor, but not the 'pill-rolling' tremor of Parkinson's; instead a coarse shake took his hand past mine as he greeted me. His feet were planted wide apart, a classic sign of the steadying compensation made when there's damage to the brain's balance-control centre, the cerebellum. And Bert had awful Paget's disease too. His calf bones were visibly distorted through his grey-flannel trousers, one bending sideways, the other forward, the 'sabre tibia' of Victorian monographs. His knuckles were lumpy with arthritis and his shoulders barely moved; he lowered himself back into his chair and pushed his chest round to bring his hand onto the table beside him to show me his drugs (paracetamol), and we sat with Queenie and talked about whether he'd like a brain scan (which he politely declined: what difference would it make?), and what else might be done. I didn't have much to offer medically.

The flat was very small and immaculate. How was he

managing? Bert told me, 'Maurice next door, he dooze the shopping,' but Bert cooked and cleaned and made the beds and looked after Queenie.

'How do you get about, Bert?' I asked.

'Mind if I show you?'

Bert got to his feet and held the arm, then the back, of his chair, then stretched his left hand out to the door frame, and next his right hand, to a rail on the wall, and took a couple of steps, then grabbed the handle of a sliding door to the tiny kitchen on the left, and pushed it forward, stepping swiftly as the door slid closed, to grab a rail again on the far side of the doorway with his other hand, and shimmied safely into the bathroom, while my palms sweated. Bert grasped the basin with both hands, and suddenly he was squatting and rising, squatting and rising, 'I dooze ten o' they,' he announced, then he held on to the basin with one hand and reached the other up just above his ear, as far as his shoulder would allow, and leaned sideways, then switched hands, and stretched the other way, 'and twenty of them ones.' Then he picked up a battered food tin, the label missing, from the edge of the bath, and lifted it, punching the tin a few inches up into the air, and he gave me a grin, eyes sparkling. 'Canadian Air Force PT. Learned it from a couple o' them boys in the war. Never missed a day.' As he spoke I realized that Bert's arms, hairy and thin, were taut with muscle.

People who exercise are less likely to fall. People who have never exercised, and start exercising, become less likely to fall. People who have fallen, and then take exercise, are less likely to fall again. We need to get moving.

The exercises that have the most effect on falling are those that contain some work on balance, like standing on one leg, and of course the best results from exercise happen in those who do a fair bit, but small steps make a difference too. It's usually a good idea to be shown how to do exercises by someone who knows what they're talking about, and to have some supervision at first, but exercise can be taken at home and can be adapted like Bert's daily routine. As Maisie, one determined woman, told me after her hip fracture, 'You don't have to "have" physio to "do" physio.' And almost everyone who takes a little exercise, even the tiniest move that makes them out of puff, feels, like Bert, the better for it, and smiles.

Our response to a fall (our own fall, or that of someone we love or care for) goes far beyond the physical, beyond bruises and blood. There's an emotional reaction too, and our behaviour – all our behaviour, that of professionals, families and patients – after a fall may define what happens next: the restoration of independence, or its loss.

Joe had fallen off his bicycle and got a humerus fracture; the X-ray showed the round head of his humerus neatly in place between shoulder blade and collarbone, but an inch further down there was a grim discontinuity: a ragged edge, and the rest of the long bone continued – not angulated, but half a bone's width out of line. That's a painful break, as pinning the pieces together has been shown to make little difference to recovery. Instead the bone is allowed to knit slowly, the arm simply supported at the wrist by a foam sling.

Joe had come to clinic a few months later and was doleful.

'I miss riding the bike, especially in this good weather,' he said.

'Why can't you ride the bike?' I asked. The foam collar and cuff were long gone. 'Is the arm still too painful?'

Joe looked surprised. 'No, they said in A & E not to ride my bike any more.'

Hang on, Joe!

'Why did you fall off the bike? What happened?'

'Well –' Joe looked up at the ceiling, replaying the day – 'I was on the back road into town, to pick up some groceries, and there was a grating left off, they must've been clearing drains, and I caught the tyre just on the edge of it.'

He banged the palm of his right hand into the side of his left, to show me how the tyre had glanced off the grating. 'Made a mess of the front wheel too.'

Oh, I was annoyed now. Eight-year-olds break their arms all the time falling off bikes, and no one tells them not to ride again. So why say that to someone who is eighty?

Joe and I had a chat. Riding his bike would be good for his legs and heart and would get him outdoors and back to meeting people. And he liked riding his bike. Joe had a plan. He'd mend the wheel and get his son to take him to the old airfield, to have a try there, back on the bike, early in the morning before the teenage novice drivers arrived to make their first kangaroo hops on the safe empty runway.

Onlookers do not like it when someone hurts themselves. Our instinct, like that of Joe's emergency doctor, is to protect. Families often feel that a fall is the tipping point: Mum has been becoming frailer; she's so unsteady, so we know something bad is going to happen – 'it's only a matter of time'. And then she has fallen, as we predicted she would, and maybe she's hurt herself badly, or maybe she was 'lucky this time', and we can't bear the idea that she is going to leave hospital, to go home once more, and we will be waiting for the same thing to happen again, or worse. And the doctor may point out that people still fall in care homes, that being in care doesn't stop you falling, but we know that in a care home Mum will be found more quickly; there'll be someone there when she's on the floor, someone to help her up or call an ambulance. But Mum listens with one ear to the discussions about her future, and she thinks of her kitchen, of the saucer under the African violet on the windowsill, and she doesn't want to go into a home.

The geriatrician – this geriatrician – does not have an answer. Each of my patients and their families must work it out, must find their own solution by triangulating the level of risk, the longing for independence and the degree of worry they can bear. I met Andy, whose mother Bridget had been a care home manager herself, and she had told him firmly, 'The minute you're worrying about me, put me in a home.'

Bridget had explained to me how she'd looked around and had found the home she wanted. 'It's a cracker, and I know what I'm talking about.'

Others feel differently. Tony said, 'If I fall, I fall, and if that's the end of me, well, that's it,' and he stuck out his lower lip and opened his hands to indicate his acceptance. Hester talked to her son and daughter, saying, 'You are not to worry about me.' But Hester's son runs a struggling business with his partner in Crete, and Hester's daughter Casey has an unforgiving boss, and a husband who is unhappy, and a child who is going through some unfathomable crisis of anxiety and identity, and how can Casey and her brother not worry about their mother, the sharp table edge, the shower tray, the top of the stairs. Often families must step back, must somehow contain their own fear and concern. We put in as good a safety net as we can afford or muster: carer visits, a lifeline pendant to call for help. After that, we must be honest about the costs – emotional rather than financial – to our own lives, and the needs of our children or spouses, and we must put boundaries around our worry and guilt, accept risk, and step aside.

*

Kathleen Graham was due to stand for the first time after her second fracture. She'd been at the community hospital a few weeks and was still not allowed to put weight through the right leg, or even bend the knee, and its every movement ached, but the left hip fracture had healed and should bear up. Until now Kathleen had been lifted from her bed to a chair by an overhead hoist. Clare the physiotherapist had been working towards this moment with her, encouraging her to strengthen the better leg as she sat, and working on her arms too, which would need to take some of her weight. Kathleen had had her hair done – on her days off one of the healthcare assistants provided a nimble shampoo and set – and was wearing another snazzy sweatshirt, this time with a kitten appliquéd to its front, a heavy navy skirt and a sturdy shoe on her left foot. Clare had brought in a different hoist, this one with a bar for Kathleen to grasp, and slings to wrap round waist and hips, to help her get up.

They were talking, heads together, as I watched from the door, but Kathleen's brow was furrowed and I could see her hand squeezing a tissue as she prepared herself, fighting with fear.

Liv poked her head in. 'How's it feeling, Kath? Bit sore?'

Kathleen looked up at us and nodded, pressing her lips together, and Liv said, 'Hang on a moment,' and Clare talked with Kathleen while we waited, showing her how the slings would help her and explaining what she needed to do to stand safely.

Liv came back, and she had a slim syringe of oral morphine liquid. 'Right-oh, Kath, time for your go-go juice.'

I watched as Clare and Liv wrapped Kath in the slings, and Kath put her tissue down on the bedside table, and placed her hands on the arms of the chair and adjusted her foot in its lace-up shoe, and the hoist whirred, and Clare knew that it was not really the fear of pain but the fear of falling that would decide the outcome, and she whispered something to Kath, and therapists sometimes do this whispering thing and the rest of us don't know what they're saying, but I think it's something about trust, about never, ever breaking that trust, and Kath pushed with her arms and straightened her leg, and up she came, standing.

Here are four things I've learned about falls. First, that they are common but are not normal, so those who have fallen deserve a proper diagnosis. Make more fuss. Second, that many (but not all) falls can be prevented by attention to detail. We should expect action. Next, that there are things any of us can do to reduce our risk of falling, namely improve our balance and strength and be proud of doing so. Finally, that a fall may have its most profound effect not through an injury but through loss of confidence. Fear of falling is real and is realistic. For my patients and their families overcoming that fear is one of the most courageous things I witness in my work.

*

You can read Prof. Close's trial here:
    https://www.ncbi.nlm.nih.gov/pubmed/10023893

You can find the National Hip Fracture Database and its leaflet, *My Hip Fracture Care: Twelve Questions to Ask*, here:
    https://www.rcplondon.ac.uk/projects/national-hip-fracture-database-nhfd

A good review of many studies examining the effects of exercise on falls is in the *British Journal of Sports Medicine* here:
    https://bjsm.bmj.com/content/51/24/1750

You may smile with this lady doing chair-based exercises:
    https://youtu.be/TnxncSUORGI

6. Not Doomed

It was June 1997 and a trickle of sweat pooled above my collarbone as I queued by the stage to ask the speaker a question. Linda Cardozo, professor in urogynaecology at King's College Hospital in London, had just delivered a well-organized lecture in which she had outlined the various surgical procedures then available to treat women who were incontinent of urine. The person in front of me was taking ages, making detailed gestures as he and the professor discussed surgical techniques. I planted my feet a little further apart. My baby was due in six weeks, and now it moved, one of its limbs pressing through the layers of my body from inside, a slow strong ripple passing just below my ribs, and I laid my hand on my bump before reaching the front of the queue. I thanked the professor for her talk.

'Professor Cardozo, may I ask what advice would you give to someone who would like to avoid needing any surgery at all?'

She looked at me, then at my bump. It was huge and even as we watched another ripple of baby limb was visible through the stretched blue fabric.

'Don't have children,' said the professor. 'And start your pelvic floor exercises when you're fourteen.'

I'm doomed. We're all doomed.

Incontinence is common. It is not normal. We are not doomed.

Around ten years ago my new colleague Bella admitted a patient to the community hospital.

'Ah, Frances,' said Bella at our weekly multidisciplinary meeting. 'I've brought her in to sort out her continence.'

I was surprised. I'd never admitted anyone to hospital in order to help their urinary incontinence. Indeed, I rarely admitted anyone electively as a planned admission; my patients all crash-landed in hospital after falls and fractures, or with pneumonia, bowel obstruction or heart failure that had suddenly worsened.

I listened as Bella explained her plan to the nurses and therapists.

'Poor woman, she's soaking. She uses loads of pads, and her skin's getting sore. She can't really move, she's got awful arthritis, and she's a *big* lady. Do you know, she has carers in six times a day, including two night visits?'

Eyebrows lifted around the table, because the maximum our local social care budget will usually allow is four visits.

Bella went on. 'They've funded it to try to keep her out of care, but it's only short term, and her skin's going to break anyway.'

I could see Henry, the staff nurse, making a note to get Frances a pressure mattress.

Bella continued. 'So here's the plan. Please can you keep a fluid intake chart? I'm not so bothered about the actual amount coming out, that's obvious, but I want to know how much she's drinking and when, and how often she's wet. And please only decaf tea and coffee. I've told her she won't taste the difference. No alcohol for now. Could you catch a pee sample and check it for sugar, and send it off to look for infection?'

Henry scribbled instructions on his handover sheet while Bella spoke.

'I've increased her heart failure meds for a while because she's pretty overloaded. I've warned her things might get worse before they get better, but while her legs are that swollen she's bound to need to pee at night – when she goes to bed the fluid from her legs all ends up in her kidneys.' Bella waved her arm to show how Frances's lower legs would move from vertical to the horizontal when she got into bed. 'I've stopped the dox-azosin; she was on it for her blood pressure but she shouldn't have been really with a heart like that, and it'll only make her bladder worse.'

I reached for a biscuit, and Bella turned to the physio Clare, and to Tony our occupational therapist.

'The really big thing is that she can't move fast enough to get to the loo. I've given her some better analgesia, a bit of morphine for now, because she's in a lot of pain: hips and knees. Obviously don't let her get constipated; I've written up the laxatives. Could we get her a commode to keep in her room so she can get to it quickly? And we really need to work on the mobility. She's got to get moving. Let me know if she needs more painkillers . . . And she might need a bed lever, I don't know, something to help her get up more quickly, whatever you think will help.'

Bella turned back to Henry. 'I know it sounds weird,' she says, 'but please could you talk to her about what she's wearing? She's got a thing about wearing woolly tights but she can't get them down in time. If she wouldn't mind staying in just her pants and maybe long socks under her skirt – no one will see.'

By now Henry's handover sheet was covered in writing, with Bella's instructions for Frances spilling up the side of the page.

'Let's see how she gets on. I've had a look and there's nothing dramatically wrong with her pelvic floor, but she might find a bit of oestrogen cream helpful. I'll have a think next week. Oh, and, by the way, she is really, really low. She hasn't left her house for three years.'

It was a masterclass. I had treated many people with continence problems, but I had never tried as hard, with as much tenacity and attention to detail, as Bella.

There are parallels between falls and continence. Each is common but not normal. The risk of each may be mitigated by action, by addressing each contributory element, so anyone who has a problem with continence deserves help. Not all falls may be prevented, nor all continence problems fixed, but things may often be made better. And, as with falls, there are things we may do for ourselves that may help.

I asked Bella for an update about the continence service she's part of. I mentioned Frances, that I've never forgotten her.

'Oh, Mrs Skelton, she was fab,' said Bella, and we looked up her letters to Frances's GP, so Bella could show me what had happened.

'She got moving, and we sorted out her heart failure,' said Bella. 'So when she went home she only needed help three times a day, and then we did a few other things and look . . .'

I read Bella's last letter.

'Mrs Skelton is now mostly dry and wears pads for confidence. She is tolerating trospium, despite some dry mouth. She has been doing pelvic floor exercises. She still has accidents but is more confident, and I was very happy to hear that she has joined a lunch club. Frances has been a star pupil.'

Continence does not fit the approach that we were taught when I was a student: that there are two sorts of urinary incontinence, one caused by an overactive bladder that you fixed with tablets, and the other, stress incontinence, which you fixed with pelvic floor exercises or surgery. Those problems do exist, often together, but continence in older people can be complicated, and usually, as with falls, needs a multifactorial approach.

I asked Bella about her continence clinic, in which she and a specialist nurse see those for whom things have become difficult.

'Here are the rules,' said Bella.

She has a kind face, a happy face. She knows how hard this can be, how impossible it might be, not just to say the words about being wet, or being unable to control bowels, but even to hear these words being said. She knows how for some people, who may have lived with incontinence for years, their pulse pounds in the ears, and vision goes blurry with shame. Somehow Bella holds eye contact, creates a layer of comfort, turns the awkwardness into something serious and funny and natural.

'I use clear words. I say "pee" or "wee", and "poo" and "vagina", and if it's a man, I say "willy" or "penis" depending what he prefers. I say "labia", or sometimes "flaps". People are uncomfortable talking about it, so we have to be tactful and kind, but you need to be able to use the right words. And I always say if you're not sure what I'm talking about, you have to tell me.'

Bella raised her eyebrows at me to check I'd understood and went on.

'I explain to people that one in three ladies over sixty-five have problems with urinary incontinence, and one in seven men. I say it really ruins people's lives. It makes them isolated and embarrassed. And I say it doesn't have to be that way. We can't always fix it, but we can almost always do something, make it better.'

As I listened to Bella I remembered that I once heard a geriatrician who worked in Bristol described as 'the one who runs towards the incontinent'. Bella was now picking up speed. She grabbed a piece of paper and outlined her knowledge.

'I say, "First, let's do all the easy things."'

Bella wrote *EASY* in big letters, then continued writing as she spoke.

'It's often a matter of thinking about the barriers to being dry. What gets between that person and the loo? What's making things worse? We talk about exactly how much they're drinking, which might be too much or sometimes not enough, because someone who knows she's going to be wet might stop drinking, but concentrated pee is irritating to the bladder and can make things worse.'

Bella had written *barriers, mobility, surroundings, clothes, equipment, intake, tea and coffee, alcohol,* all the things she had done for Frances, the things she does for all her patients, the things she calls 'easy', but that are too easy to overlook.

'You've got to do the basics first. You've got to think about mechanism, and it's likely to be several things going on at once. Check for infection, check for sugar, do a bladder scan.'

Bella was explaining that incontinence of urine in men or women may be due paradoxically to a bladder that doesn't empty; it fills and fills, and eventually overflows in an uncontrollable way. In men that's often due to a big benign prostate gland; in women, especially those who are very frail, or have broken a hip, or who have dementia, it may be due to constipation. Bladder scans, to make sure incontinence isn't due to an over-flowing bladder, are quick and easy, and every ward and nursing home should have a scanner but doesn't.

Bella wrote *BLADDER SCAN*, then drew a line, and wrote a new heading.

'Then it's going to be either pelvic floor stuff, or drugs for an overactive bladder, or usually both.'

She drew a line and wrote *PELVIC FLOOR*.

'The pelvic floor, the muscles that hold everything in place and squeeze the bladder neck so it doesn't leak. It's sometimes a good idea to try oestrogen creams or pessaries. If everything's a bit dry, which just happens when we're older, it'll be better for being given a bit of oestrogen. Lots of older women get a bit sore underneath and think that's normal but it isn't. And there's some evidence that topical oestrogen can help reduce urine infections too. Plush is lush.'

Bella smiled as she wrote, and continued. 'And you've got to get those muscles as strong as they can be. Lots of people, especially older ladies, are a bit lost when it comes to even knowing what their pelvic floor is. I try to get people to see Sue downstairs in physio. She has them cracking walnuts before they know it.'

I went to see Sue in her consulting room, with its posters and models of bladders and bottoms, and told her about Bella's nut-cracking commendation. Sue blushed, but only at being paid a compliment, not at the subject. She is a continence physio and explains in clear, unembarrassed language how to work out what and where a pelvic floor is, and she teaches women – and men – how to strengthen it.

Sue explained, 'I don't know about being able to crack nuts. But I do know that older people can do well with pelvic floor exercises. To be honest they've never been shown before, so it's nice to know what to do. And they've often got time to do them.'

'What about surgery?' I asked Sue, and she pulled a face.

'I think sometimes people are pushed into that too quickly. They need to get a proper chance at exercise first. They need to be told what to do by someone who knows what they're on about. It can be hard to work out how to do pelvic floor exercises from a leaflet.'

I listened to another physiotherapist, Elaine Miller, describing on *Woman's Hour* exactly how to do these exercises. Elaine is great. She has performed her explanation at the Edinburgh festival, a pelvic-floor show, and right now she's on an education mission in Australia ('I'm trying not to say "Down Under"'). Elaine got the giggles – not embarrassed giggles, but joyous giggles – as she explained on national radio what we need to do.

'You have to sort out your breath. If you sigh out first, it's much easier to get your pelvic floor to contract. So take a deep breath, then sigh out, then imagine that you're trying to hold in a fart.'

There's a nervous hoot from Jenni Murray.

Elaine is undeterred. 'Think about, you are in a lift, with people you really don't want to embarrass yourself in front of – your boss, your mother-in-law, your secret crush. What you feel in your bum is a squeeze and a lift, when you imagine yourself trying to hold something in, and that's your pelvic floor. So breathe in, sigh out, squeeze and lift, and hold it for ten seconds. But you've got to keep breathing at the same time.'

Elaine explains how we each need to do that 'squeeze and lift' ten times, no buttock clenching – 'Instead you're holding your bits up off your gusset.' Then we can do ten 'quick flicks', a quick contraction and relax. As Elaine explains, the pelvic floor must have the strength to hold on, if we need a pee and there's nowhere to go, but also needs to be able to contract quickly if we laugh or cough.

I took no notice of Professor Cardozo's advice at the time. I had two more children, and got very busy, and exercises seemed silly and irrelevant. My friends and I joked about how we would never again be able to leap about on a trampoline, and we crossed our legs, subtly we thought, when we sneezed. And I turned fifty and took up a fitness class, an enlivening boot camp on a Monday evening, and the instructor would demand star jumps, and I could see certain women catch one another's eye, and we would substitute some other movement, less calamitous. My friend Clo read me the Riot Act, and made me download the NHS Squeezy app on to my phone for £2.99, and that app bossed me around, reminding me to do those pelvic floor exercises, and I had to programme it not to go off in the middle of a ward round, but find instead better times, maybe sitting in the car gathering my thoughts for the day or in an X-ray meeting. And even then I contrived to ignore it until one day I got fed up with myself for doling out advice to others that I didn't follow myself, and I made a plan and stuck to it, my pelvic floor equivalent of a 'couch to 5k', just two minutes at a time, three times each day, and, believe me, it helps.

Bella and I talked about surgery too.

'Surgery is right for some people. Sometimes, with a big prolapse, they're just so damaged, they're never going to come right with exercise alone. But prolapse surgery can make things worse; you want to try a decent pessary, properly fitted, first. If that doesn't help the continence, surgery probably won't either.'

Bella was a member of the most recent NICE committee reviewing surgery for urinary incontinence in women and has scrutinized every piece of evidence and is aware of the painful testimony from those who have been harmed by surgical mesh procedures as well as the happy stories from those whose lives have been positively transformed. She went on, 'Surgery now is more complex and recovery can be longer, because the mesh and tape operations aren't allowed. And that's sometimes just not a valid option for frailer older women.'

I thought back to Frances and the various things Bella tried. One of Bella's lectures starts with a cartoon – a harassed-looking receptionist has picked up the phone, and says 'National Continence Helpline, can you hold?'

'What about bladder retraining?' I asked Bella, and

she sighed. The ageing bladder can get ratty; it doesn't wait to fill up before it wants to be emptied. It's not just age – it can happen to younger people too. Other things like Parkinson's, stroke, MS, make an overactive bladder worse. It doesn't seem fair. Bladder retraining is a technique that can help those whose bladder is overactive. It involves consciously ignoring the desire to pee, making the bladder wait for a few extra minutes each time, so that it becomes more used to filling up properly before demanding to be emptied.

Bella explained the difficulty. 'Retraining really can work for those with an overactive bladder, but it depends on the underlying diagnoses and it's sometimes easier for younger people. It depends on asking someone to wait, to make their bladder hold on, and that can be a real challenge. Fifteen minutes of hanging on can be impossible. If I do suggest it, I set the bar low. I might suggest they try waiting just an extra thirty seconds, and build up from here, just to one minute perhaps, but even that can be too much. With things like Parkinson's disease the bladder gets so trigger happy, they often just can't hang on at all. For some people with an overactive bladder after we've tried everything else we may have to try the drugs.'

Bella wrote *DRUGS*.

'The drugs can sometimes help. If we're going down the anticholinergic line – tolterodine, solifenacin, trospium, whatever – I now always, always warn people about the side effects: dry mouth, dry eyes, constipation.'

The anticholinergics are a group of drugs used to

treat an overactive bladder. Their side effects are important, and I talk about them in Chapter 7.

Bella continued her explanation. 'And I say we just don't know about their effect on the brain. We know that it's possible that when they're used for a long time, maybe over several years, these drugs might affect brain function. Maybe avoid them altogether in someone who is at risk of developing dementia, although that is an important discussion to have . . . Weigh up the risk versus the benefit. And I say for heaven's sake don't take them if they're not working. Give them, say, six, eight weeks. At most three months. People often only get one appointment in a continence service so there's no follow-up to check the drug's making any difference. The drugs make no difference for more than half of people. I say they must make a second appointment with a GP or practice nurse who can stop the prescription if it's not helping. Or you can just stop taking them, but make sure you've told the GP you've stopped so they know to stop issuing the tablets.'

Bella added the names of a few more of the anticholinergic drugs. There are many.

'If one doesn't work, and someone's really having a bad time, sometimes it's worth playing around, trying different ones. If none help, I might try mirabegron; it sometimes helps, but you can't use it in anyone with high blood pressure.'

Mirabegron's a drug in a different class, not an anticholinergic. Again, it makes a difference for some people.

Bella and I talked about those with dementia, who may become incontinent because they don't remember that they need to go or what the social rules are about where we pee and poo. Bella was clear. 'It's not fair to forget that people who have dementia can become incontinent for all the same reasons as people who don't have dementia. So you mustn't just assume it's dementia if there's new incontinence. For example, some of the medicines used to treat dementia can act to make people incontinent, like donepezil or rivastigmine. And you still need to do the easy things like excluding infection and constipation and overflow. But once you've done that, it is tricky, and it's kind that someone should be offered regular visits to the toilet, make it as easy as possible, but it's still difficult to fix, and chances are we'll have to work on "contain" rather than cure.'

As well as referring people to Sue for advice, Bella runs a joint clinic with Edie. Edie is a continence nurse. *The* continence nurse. It takes ages to track her down. She is busy.

'Do you enjoy it?' I ask her.

'It's a lovely job. You can make a difference. People are so shy, some of them have had problems for years, and there's that stigma, about old ladies smelling of wee, and sometimes I have to say, "Do you know, whatever happens you don't have to smell of wee?" People's lives are so badly affected and it doesn't need to be like that.'

Edie reiterates Bella's advice about the easy things, and adds, 'And try to stop drinking three hours before bed. It's amazing how people still have a cup of tea or Horlicks or whatever last thing, and when you're older that means you'll be up in the night.'

I ask Edie what other things people might find surprising, about how their bottoms work.

'I spend a lot of time advising people about bowels too, because so many people get constipation, and they usually know about diet, to try prunes and apricots, but maybe they don't realize about checking through their tablets to see if any are making things worse and asking if they can be changed. And something that sounds silly but makes a difference is how you sit on the loo. You need your feet on a firm surface, so you can lean forward and tilt your pelvis a bit. It can make a real difference to put your feet on a stool in front of the loo, so you're in more of a squatting position. And if you're a little lady and you go into a care home, you know, with raised toilet seats, you might not be able to even reach the floor; your feet are dangling, which is no good. So you need to be given something to put your feet on.'

Edie and I talk about some of the specialist treatments that can help – Botox injections to relax a bladder, sacral nerve stimulators for some people with faecal incontinence to wake up a bumhole muscle that is intact but weak, and she points out that these are helpful for some but that many people, especially those who are more frail, don't want to try those treatments.

Edie goes on. 'What I'd like people to know most is that they're not alone and it's not their fault, and we can usually help. And I know it sounds defeatist, but even if we can't stop you being leaky, the containment is so much better than it was even a few years ago. Pads are better designed, more comfortable. They hold more, and don't smell. I think it's reassuring to know that.'

Continence services are widely available across the UK. All are accessible via a referral from a GP. Many services allow people to refer themselves by email or by telephone. It's a step worth taking.

Mrs Everton stands at the end of Dennis's bed, her hands on her hips. She's wearing a cream polo neck and brown trousers, and her polo neck is snug so I can see the indentations at her shoulders of the wide straps of her bra, which is a hardworking garment, and Mrs Everton looks proud and angry and worried and exhausted all at the same time, and she has been in and out of this hospital almost every day for over two weeks while Dennis has got first better, then worse, then better again, working his way through a list of medical events to add to his previous strokes, his heart failure, his prostate problems. Dennis has been declared 'medically fit for discharge', although Mrs Everton wasn't impressed when the therapist told her this, and Mrs Everton has said that Dennis 'isn't fit for a haircut, anyone could see that,' and that she supposes it'll all be down to her again now to look after Dennis, but that she wants him home, any road, because he'll be happier there. To which Dennis has nodded and curled his good left hand into a thumbs up, and his bad old right hand, screwed in a ball, has rubbed itself on his chest as it tried too to convey enthusiasm for this plan.

'But, Dr Lucy, you're going to have to do something about his water trouble,' says Mrs Everton, and she's right, because to accompany Dennis's pneumonia, his swallowing problems, his out-of-kilter kidneys and unaccountably swollen wrist, Dennis's waterworks have played a low rumbling continuo of trouble, with soaked pads and wet beds, which Dennis can't talk about because Dennis can't talk about anything since the last stroke. And these wet beds cause him to look out of the window at the big soft leaves of the Indian bean tree when the young HCAs come in to change him, and take off his pyjamas, bottom and top, both wet, and pad and sheets, all wet. And I know this was a problem too before Dennis came in, and everything has been assessed and tried. Occasionally Dennis's bladder stops working altogether because his prostate has got big, even though he had surgery years ago, but most of the time it is just bad-tempered and impatient and gives Dennis no respite from its demands, which he cannot meet.

Dennis has been on finasteride, a drug I like a lot, even though it takes a while to work – up to six months and beyond for maximum effect. It's a hormone treatment that blocks a potent form of testosterone in the prostate, causing it eventually to shrink, and improving flow. Finasteride seems to have some protective effect against prostate cancer, and although one might think that a drug that interferes with testosterone might damage libido or cause problems with erections, this seems to affect fewer men than one might expect – around one in a hundred in some studies, up to 15% in another, although in that study the placebo drug caused similar problems and we know that a man's ability to have an erection is controlled by a great deal more than mechanics alone. But Dennis has been on finasteride for years and it's not working any more, and he can't take alpha blockers because they make his blood pressure go too low, so he gets light-headed when he stands up, which he can barely do at the best of times, and he can't take the bladder-calming medicines because his bladder huffily stops emptying altogether on those, and while he's been in hospital we've tried Conveens, which are like a condom with tubing attached, but they haven't worked for Dennis, slipping off within minutes. At present Dennis has a proper catheter in place, and Mrs Everton says that's made all the difference, and he slept better last night, and please could he just come home with that catheter? So we have a chat about the risks of infection, which are real, because bacteria creep up a catheter no matter how fastidious you are about keeping it clean, and the risks thus include the possibility of life-threatening sepsis, but Mrs Everton says she thinks Dennis will take that risk, because this is no life, there's no dignity, to which Dennis again nods vigorously, so the catheter is a fine plan, and Mrs Everton readies herself to learn how to look after Dennis's catheter, to build on her knowledge of his tablets, and the pressure mattress upon which he sleeps at home, and the turning frame she uses to help him out of bed, and the thickening powder she adds to his drinks, to get them to exactly syrup consistency, and I want to hug Mrs Everton, but she is a dignified woman and still has her hands on her hips, so I say instead, 'Do you mind, Mrs Everton, if I say that you are doing a great job? And you are doing all the right things for this husband of yours.' Mrs Everton gives a sniff and a nod, and turns to get a clean shirt out of the bag that she has brought in for Dennis.

Bella and I looked at the rest of Frances's letters. She lived for only another eighteen months after leaving the community hospital before she died of the heart failure that was part of the problem when she came in. But she went on living in her own home until her final short admission to hospital, and there's a letter from one of the heart failure nurses that mentions how much Frances enjoys the lunch club, and I suspect that perhaps sorting out Frances's continence made more difference than anything else to her happiness in the last part of her life.

*

Age UK has a good page explaining continence problems:

    https://www.ageuk.org.uk/information-advice/health-wellbeing/conditions-illnesses/incontinence/#

7. Goldilocks Medicine

Dee Mangin is a GP from New Zealand. In a video clip she made in 2017, she talked about a seventy-year-old woman, who had five common conditions: high blood pressure (most people over seventy have that), diabetes, arthritis, osteoporosis and COPD (chronic obstructive pulmonary disease, which used to be called smoker's lung or bronchitis and emphysema). Dee explained that if her patient was treated for each of these conditions according to current guidance, she would take nineteen doses of twelve different medications at five different times of day. Dee next observed that this would give rise to at least sixteen possible harmful interactions; either the drugs may interact with one another, or a drug that improved one condition may inadvertently worsen something else. She went on to say that what looked like good care, if you considered only single diseases, could result in 'meaningfully worse care' for the individual.

Early in her career Dee Mangin had observed the negative effects of medication in her older patients. She became worried about the direct harms of some medicines and their interactions, and about the psychological downside of people being prescribed medicines for conditions that were not yet causing symptoms and that may or may not cause future harm. She became concerned too that using preventive medicines in older age may mean simply exchanging one risk for another – preventing heart attacks using statins in very old age may mean her patient became more likely to die of cancer. It's not that statins cause cancer, it's just that we all must die of something. Iona Heath and the late Kieran Sweeney are two British GPs with whom Mangin wrote a powerful article in the *BMJ* in 2007, examining the perverse drivers of 'preventive' prescribing. They concluded, 'By providing treatments designed to prevent particular diseases we may be selecting for another cause of death unknowingly, and certainly without the patient's informed consent. This is fundamentally unethical and undermines the principle of respect for autonomy.'

The patient Dee Mangin spoke about in her video was a young woman, only seventy: the lecture was illustrated by a photo of a chirpy-looking lady doing an exercise class in a swimming pool.

I thought about Dee's lecture while I sat in an outpatient clinic reading a GP referral letter about Peggy. The clinic was in one of our small community hospitals. I could hear a blackbird and a low drone from a lawnmower on the far side of the building. The window was open and the vertical blinds were tapping together in an early-summer breeze.

Peggy had had a couple of falls and was becoming weak. The letter described her breathlessness, poor sleep

and loss of appetite. Her GP listed several conditions –
Peggy had type 2 diabetes, and cardiac failure caused by
stiffening of her heart muscle. She'd had a small stroke at
some point and had broken her wrist six years previously. Peggy had leg ulcers and arthritis, and a history of
high blood pressure. She was eighty-six. A list of Peggy's
medicines was appended. I rubbed my nose as I read.

I looked through Peggy's blood results, and the discharge summary from a week-long hospital stay after
the most recent fall. I read old letters from cardiology
and the stroke clinic, then went to the waiting room to
find her.

At Exeter University a team led by Professor David
Melzer have studied how we collect diseases as we get
older. It becomes unusual to have just one condition: illnesses come along like buses. For example, over 90% of
people who have dementia also have something else
wrong. Almost everyone with heart failure, like Peggy,
has at least one other chronic condition: in those with
heart failure who are also over eighty-five years old most
will have at least three or four other diseases to contend
with. A quarter will have more than five. Diseases gang
up as we age; some share causes, or cause one another,
and the number of chronic conditions we have increases
decade on decade (until we find the centenarians, who
are the survivors, and often have very few diagnoses. As
a colleague observed, 'Have you noticed how light their
notes are?').

*

Peggy was sitting in a high-backed green chair, solidly filling the seat, her broad hips stretching her burgundy wool skirt. Her hair was bouffant, and she was wearing a neat dark green blazer with a golden fleur-de-lis brooch. She gave an anxious smile as I spoke her name, and her husband leaped up to put her walking frame in front of her. Peggy rocked gently back and forth a couple of times, before pushing herself up using the arms of the chair. There was a moment of peril as she let go of the chair and grabbed for the frame, like a trapeze artist stretching for her partner's rescuing grasp, then she leaned forward, crossing her arms on the frame while she took a couple of deep breaths before straightening up for the long, long walk to the consulting room. It's eight metres.

I walked beside her and asked about her journey – she stood still for a moment to tell me about Joe's good driving, and how he had made sure they had plenty of time to get here.

'You found a good husband,' I said, and Peggy agreed. 'He does everything now. I'd be lost without him.'

At the door of the room I turned to greet Joe; he was towing a tartan shopping trolley and carrying Peggy's handbag, and was dapper in his grey tweed suit.

In the short walk from a waiting area to a consulting room those who attend appointments with geriatricians tell us more about themselves than they might realize. Peggy had taken more than five seconds to walk four metres; this is an indicator of frailty. I could see that she would not pass a 'timed up and go' test – even with her frame she would not be able to stand, walk three metres and back, and sit, within twelve seconds. That's another frailty sign, and told me too that she was at increased risk of falling. In order to answer my question about her journey Peggy had to stop walking, and being unable to walk and talk at the same time is a well-studied marker of falls risk. There are many scales on which geriatricians can measure frailty. Before we got to the consulting-room door I knew that Peggy scored at least five on one of them, a PRISMA-7 scale, based on her age and health problems, her use of a walking frame and the help she needed each day – a total of three or more indicates frailty. And her GP's computer system had already done the work, totting up Peggy's diagnosis list, using an electronic Frailty Index, the eFI, to declare that she had frailty, and that her level of frailty was severe.

We sat together and went through Peggy's problems and the things she'd tried so far. Her breathing was better than it had been when she was in hospital, but she still felt exhausted and couldn't walk beyond the garden path. They'd had a stair lift installed, and the practice nurses had been tending her leg ulcers for over a year. I looked at Peggy's blood pressure, taken while she'd been waiting, and listened to her heart and breathing, dropping the weighty end of my stethoscope like a plumb line down inside her blouse and wriggling it as low as I could before being thwarted by stern corsetry. Her legs were equally inaccessible, with thick tan stockings stretched tightly over carefully applied compression bandages.

'May I have a look at your medicines?' I asked, and Peggy looked across to Joe, who brought forward the shopping trolley. He delved, and produced an old ice-cream tub, its lid held in place by an elastic band. Out came another ice-cream tub, then a shortbread biscuit tin, and from the bottom of the trolley two big pots of emollient creams. I spread the medicines out on the desk and watched Peggy's face. She looked despondent.

'That's a lot of tablets,' I said.

'She's rattling, doctor,' Joe told me.

Peggy joined in. 'We say we could open a pharmacy.'

Iona Heath, by then president of the Royal College of GPs, observed in an essay in 2010: 'All clinicians caring for older people have the experience of treating one disease process, only for another to take its place; and the more diseases that coexist, the greater the hazards of overtreatment and polypharmacy, and the more the challenges of daily life become a struggle.'

Peggy, Joe and I looked at the medicines on the desk, and I divided the cartons up into three loose sections. Polypharmacy is the use of five or more medicines. The patient I had seen immediately before Peggy had been taking nine; the one before that, twelve. Peggy was taking fifteen.

Since 2007, when she wrote that article with Heath and Sweeney about preventive treatments, Dee Mangin has devoted much of her career to working out how best to help people make informed decisions about their medicine – how to provide the autonomy that these three GPs felt was so lacking. Mangin became a professor of primary care in Otago in New Zealand, and later moved to McMaster University in Canada, where her research includes polypharmacy. Mangin's group have developed a project called TAPER, Team Approach to Polypharmacy Evaluation and Reduction; it was the launch of that project I had watched on her video clip. And most importantly for Mangin the key member of the polypharmacy project team is the patient.

'OK, Peggy, let's start here.' I lifted two cartons from the left-hand pile. 'Do you find some of these helpful?'

She looked at them and nodded. 'Those ones are good.'

'Right, so we'll keep them.'

Peggy smiled. I moved the paracetamol and laxatives back into an ice-cream tub, and picked up her water tablet, furosemide.

'If you stopped your water tablet, I reckon your legs would swell up and you'd get more breathless pretty quickly.'

Joe agreed. 'That's what happened when you were in the hospital last time.'

So I put the furosemide back into the tub, and chose another carton, saying, 'These ones are keeping your thyroid in order; you could miss them out for a while but if you left them off for long you would start feeling more tired and slowed up.' I put the thyroxine with the other 'keepers'.

We'd done the easy bit. The tablets that made Peggy feel better today were safely stowed away in the ice-cream tub. There were still many boxes on the desk. Her fifteen prescriptions meant that Peggy had been taking seventeen tablets every morning, with a bonus pill on Sundays, another three at lunch, two at teatime, and eight before bed. The next two heaps were going to need more thinking about.

Frailty has become the subject of much research in geriatric medicine, and to many its implications must seem obvious. Since its inception as a specialty geriatricians have known they are caring for the most vulnerable, the Ming vases, old, precious and fragile – but it's only in recent years that this vulnerability has been given a formal label. Frailty now has a definition – the British Geriatrics Society calls it 'a distinctive health state related to the ageing process in which multiple body systems gradually lose their in-built reserves'. If something bad happens, a person with frailty is less likely to recover. Much research is dedicated to the hunt for ways in which frailty can be prevented or improved; it is not felt to be an inevitable part of ageing. Not everyone who is old has frailty, and young people can have frailty – but many people with frailty are very old and have numerous conditions.

If we looked at each of their medical problems separately, people with frailty might seem to need *more* tablets so that we might reduce the risk of their conditions getting worse. But many drug trials only look at what happens to one disease; they don't always look at all-cause mortality, and they don't consider the complexity of having several conditions at once, the dangers of drug interactions, and the sheer burden of taking multiple medicines.

Peggy, Joe and I looked at the next pile of medicines. People with frailty, like Peggy, are more likely to fall or to get delirious when they are ill or to be admitted to hospital, and they are substantially more likely to die within a given time frame. They take longer to recover from operations, or don't recover at all. And people with frailty are much more likely to develop side effects of drugs.

Into the middle heap I had put the medicines that were meant to be making Peggy feel better, but were less likely to be working or more likely to give side effects. I picked up another tablet, tolterodine; it's one of a group of medicines (sometimes called anticholinergics) designed to calm an irritable bladder. These drugs work. They work for one in nine people, who notice the benefit, and are relieved.

'Um . . . Peggy, this one's for your waterworks. Do you ever get caught short on the way to the toilet?'

She shifted in her chair. 'A fair bit,' she said.

I asked if she used a pad, and she explained that she did, and that she looked out for where the toilets were when they went shopping.

'Do you reckon this tablet's made any difference?' I asked.

'I wouldn't say so,' she told me, and looked to Joe, who shook his head.

'Do you ever get a dry mouth?'

Peggy widened her eyes at me, and she puffed out a breath. 'Always.'

This is madness! These drugs work for around one in nine people. Eight out of nine people taking bladder-calming tablets get no noticeable benefit and are simply at risk of their common side effects: dry eyes, dry mouth, constipation. Worryingly these side effects are likely to include a reduction in brain function, difficult to measure but real (the chemical they target, acetylcholine, is essential for cognition. Most dementia drugs work by boosting its levels. The drugs to calm a bladder have the opposite effect, blocking acetylcholine, and the evidence is mounting that these drugs, together with a wide variety of other drugs that have incidental 'anticholinergic' properties, such as some antidepressants, are, in the long term, not good for the brain).

'I wonder if it's worth taking a break from this one. Would you like to stop it for a few weeks, and see what happens? If the waterworks get worse, you can decide whether you want to go back on it again, or we might try some other things.'

I wrote *HOLIDAY* across the tolterodine box and gave it back to Peggy. We were going through these medications with a fine-tooth comb; everything on her prescription list must earn its place. Peggy, Joe and I were deprescribing together and it was going to get complicated.

We set up a 'bin pile', and into this we put Peggy's angina tablet, nicorandil; it reduces angina attacks, but is now recognized for sometimes causing ulceration (in the mouth, around the bottom, throughout the gut) and for preventing wound healing. Peggy's leg ulcers would never heal while she was on nicorandil, and in any case it turned out she hadn't had angina for years or maybe at all; she and Joe thought it might have been indigestion. Angina's important, but it's also a label that gets attached easily when someone's had chest pain for other reasons. In addition, people with true angina don't always have angina forever. It often disappears completely after a heart attack, or after a procedure like a stent. And in very old or frail people angina may go away simply because they can no longer exert themselves.

Now we turned to Peggy's diabetes tablets. When she was collected by the ambulance after her latest fall the paramedics recorded a low sugar level. Another blood test done by her GP had shown that Peggy's sugar control was good – too good.

People with diabetes are encouraged to keep their glucose levels between narrow goalposts, because high sugar levels slowly but inexorably damage the delicate lining of blood vessels, and in turn the organs supplied by those precious little arteries become unhappy. Kidneys shrink and harden; vessels in the back of the eye stiffen and leak; nerve endings wither; calf muscles ache for more oxygen; and toes may blacken as their supply lines dwindle. But this damage happens over decades, not over months or even a few years. In young people – in their fifties or sixties say – good control of diabetes buys extra years of active life. The effort they put into watching what they eat, and taking the right tablets, and endless blood tests, pays off. But for older people danger may lurk in control that is too good. Older people with diabetes are at more risk of drug-induced hypoglycaemia (low sugar), which is associated with falls, and can cause lasting damage to brain function. In the USA there are now more emergency admissions for hypos due to over-treated diabetes in the over-sixty-fives than for hyperglycaemia. Hypos are even more common in those over seventy-five, and for the very oldest patients with type 2 diabetes there's no long-term reward for avoiding moderately high sugars. Provided she was not thirsty or peeing lots, I would not be too worried about Peggy getting high sugar levels – in very old age, and with other problems going on, it's the low levels, the hypos, that are more likely to cause trouble.

I put one box of Peggy's diabetes tablets in the bin pile and halved the dose of the other. We would need to agree – with Peggy, with her GP and her practice nurse – a change of her diabetes goalposts, to concentrate on ensuring that her levels did not make her feel unwell now, in the present, rather than aiming for an unattainable nirvana of metabolic perfection, which may cause her harm.

So far Peggy, Joe and I had whittled down the tablets that weren't working, or that had damaging side effects. We had adjusted the tablets that had been doing a good job in the past, but that now needed reducing as the goals of Peggy's treatment had changed.

In the maelstrom of hurried appointments with different doctors and complicated drug regimes it's easy for drugs to be started, less easy for them to be stopped. Peggy and I needed time to unpick the story, to pin down a diagnosis that no longer existed, or which was wrong in the first place. Time to apprehend a tablet with too many side effects or that wasn't doing its job. Time for Peggy and me to consider her needs and priorities, which would change just as inevitably as her face gathered lines.

Time, though, would not be all we needed.

Peggy, Joe and I turned our attention at last to the third pile, the one on the right. These were not making Peggy feel better at all – they were not meant to. They were there to reduce the risk of some future problem. Here sat her statin, her aspirin, a couple of blood pressure tablets, her osteoporosis medicines. Now we would need to think hard and share some uncertainties.

When I'm trying to work out what to do with Peggy's medicines I need to be honest about her prospects. Peggy's life expectancy should be around six more years – about half of eighty-six-year-old women make it to ninety-two and beyond. But that's an average, and includes all the fit eighty-six-year-olds who are rushing around doing Pilates and driving 'old people' to appointments. At eighty-six *and* with severe frailty Peggy's prospects narrow; realistically her life expectancy might be three years. Her dodgy heart blurs the picture still further. Heart failure has a gloomy outlook overall, but it's unpredictable, with periods of stability punctuated by sudden severe episodes, which makes it harder to guess what's round the corner. Peggy's limited life expectancy presents a paradox; she may not live long enough to benefit from some of the medicines that are designed to improve long-term outlook. But if she doesn't take them, perhaps her life will be shortened.

The further paradox with the medicines designed to reduce future risk, is the concern expressed by those three thoughtful GPs in 2007: that we may simply be switching one mode of death for another. In younger people treatment may prevent a premature death, but in much older people another illness will inevitably, and perhaps soon, come forward to take the place of the one we have averted. Heath's 2010 essay was titled 'What Do We Want to Die From?', and geriatricians and GPs know exactly what she means – the price for treating your high blood pressure may be an increased risk of your hip breaking. Statins reduce deaths from heart attacks and strokes, but avoiding death from one disease means we must die of something else. How might we best decide what to do? Can current research tell us the answer?

People like Peggy don't get into trials of medication. Older people, especially those with frailty, are hard to study. They may be taking other medicines that interfere with the trial drug, or they develop other illnesses during the research, which means they may drop out of the trial too early; they might even die of something that is not of interest to the researcher. They may struggle to come to the research appointments because they're not very mobile, or maybe because their spouse gets ill and can't bring them. Older people are much more prone to side effects, so it's easier to run a trial in younger, fitter people, who have perhaps only one or two conditions, and whose brains, livers and kidneys are resilient. (Even in her forties Caitlin Moran noticed the diminution in her liver function, and compared a noisome hangover to those of her youth, lamenting that back then 'I had the rosy, capable liver of a child.') The truth is, if you were a pharmaceutical company keen to demonstrate that your drug was safe, you wouldn't want to try it out in the group of patients who are most likely to develop a problem.

Thus for decades the over-eighties were systematically excluded from drug trials. In the great studies of drugs for heart failure towards the end of the last century the average participant was in his youthful mid-sixties (and was a man). Even now, when drug companies are keener to include old people in trials, they keep the

exclusion criteria tight. The over-eighties are theoretic-
ally allowed to join in, but there's always a clause that
allows researchers to disbar those who may prove prob-
lematic: people living in care homes, for example, and
those with other important conditions like kidney
disease or dementia, or people whom the researchers
consider 'unreliable'. When you look closely the older
people in most drug trials are a select group, fitter than
their peers, and with only one or two medical problems. Peggy would not be one of them.

This leaves doctors in an awkward position. Should
we blithely extrapolate the results of studies done mostly
on people in their sixties, with one or two conditions, to
those in their eighties and nineties, with five or six? We
don't want to deny older people effective treatments, yet
we are not sure whether they *are* effective treatments for
these complicated patients.

The final paradox with prescribing preventive medicines for people like Peggy lies in the downside of drugs.
Most drugs are very safe. Side effects are not ubiquitous,
and are not usually life threatening. However, side effects
do happen, and can be severe, and older people with or
without frailty are more prone to them. Arguments rage
as to precisely how often drugs cause hospital admissions because the data is hard to collect. The statistics
may record someone's admission as being due to 'acute
kidney injury', for example, but it's not clear whether it
was the new blood pressure drug or the bout of dehy-
drating gastroenteritis that pushed those ageing kidneys

over the edge – most likely it was a bit of both. And some side effects are subtle – a drug may have slow, cumulative effects on brain function, or cause muscle weakness or bone thinning or reduced absorption of important vitamins, which are difficult to detect. Yet I need to maintain my balance. After a ward round sorting out a big bleed in someone who has been taking a blood thinner, and the next patient, who has had a life-changing fall because tablets pushed their blood pressure too low, and the person after that, who has terrifying confusion caused by their sodium plummeting due to another medication, I feel enraged by the medication-related misery I have witnessed, and I struggle to remember that this morning I did not see the stroke that didn't happen, the heart attack averted.

James liked his meds. He presented me with a neat list – it ran to a second page, and James had typed up the indication for each medicine alongside the doses and times. *To prevent stroke*, read one; *to prevent heart attack*; *to prevent stomach ulcer*. I raised my eyebrows, but he told me proudly, 'I have an excellent general practitioner,' and I didn't feel I should pickily point out that none of these drugs actually 'prevent' anything, they just reduce the risk of one thing or another, usually by a small amount, while at the same time slightly increasing the risk of something else. I suspected James was aware of this, but he was happy with the balance of benefits and risks represented by his carefully typed list. James felt he was being well looked after, which he was, and none of his medications was visibly causing harm, and he was contented. I left his list well alone.

Many other people, though, are not like James. Many of my patients have serious misgivings about their medications, but they gather a selection of pills each morning into a cupped hand, hustling them down with a swig of tea and shaking their head as they wonder what was that for? And for those who are unable to make their own decisions families and care home staff place a cluster of pills on a saucer or into a little plastic pot, and a husband or a daughter-in-law or a carer coaxes and cajoles, and they worry about what will happen if the pills are not taken, and they worry about whether the pills are doing any good, or are causing harm.

The third group of Peggy's medicines still sitting on the desk may or may not be causing any physical side effects, yet were contributing to her feeling downcast. Many people are hesitant about questioning their doctor about the purpose of their medicines, and they either struggle manfully on, like Peggy, despite a feeling of unease, or they adopt techniques to avoid the tablets about which they feel most wary. Boxes of medicines are hidden at the back of drawers; pills are slipped down the side of an armchair, folded into bedsheets, tucked under a half-eaten biscuit. Each of these is a sad sight, such a waste of effort and money, and each points to a relationship that is a little broken, between a doctor, steadfastly prescribing in accordance with guidelines, and a person who is unable for one reason or another to tell their doctor that they will not or cannot take the tablets.

So, the next thing we need after time is honesty. Doctors need to be honest about the limitations of our knowledge about what works and what doesn't in people who are older, and especially in those who are frail and have several conditions and maybe do not have very long to live. Doctors need to be honest about the fact that reducing the risk of one condition may not lengthen life, but will simply exchange one cause of death for another. We must be honest about the fact that many medications probably aren't making a great deal of difference. But patients and their families need to be honest too about what they feel about their medicines. We all need to be able to talk together about the purpose of medicines, and that means being honest that for many of my patients their hope may not be simply to lengthen an already long life, but rather to improve and preserve its quality.

Here we come to the last pieces of the prescribing jigsaw. Sorting out polypharmacy is complicated and needs to be done by those taking the tablets, or their families and carers, working closely with doctors who have had plenty of training, supported by knowledgeable pharmacists and good IT systems that can spot errors and subtle interactions. We need time to do it well. We need honesty between patients and doctors, about what matters most.

There's a final barrier to getting it right. I'd been at a

training day with GPs. We'd been discussing polypharmacy and the difficulty of making good shared decisions.
I'd talked about the balancing act involved in decisions
about blood thinners, anticoagulants used when the
heart is in an irregular rhythm called atrial fibrillation
(AF) in order to reduce the risk of a stroke. The problem is that anticoagulants reduce the risk of a blockage
in an artery but simultaneously increase the risk of
bleeding.

Maarike was frowning. She is a GP, Dutch, jolly and
outspoken, and right now she was exasperated.

'Look,' said Maarike. 'I hef this old man, nice old
man, liffs in a care home. And he hass big, big nose
bleeds, all the time. He's going up and down to the hospital, blood transfusions, and in the endt, I say, "Jacky,
this is too much for you, let us stop this blood thinnink
tablet, what do you think?" And he says, "Yes, good
plan, Dr Maarike." And we stop the blood thinner, and
a month or so later he hass this big stroke, and he lives a
few weeks more, in a bad state, and then he is dead, and
I know . . .'

Maarike stopped and looked at the ceiling of the audi-
torium, and even though she was speaking in an echoing
room, surrounded by people who maybe did not know
her, and who never knew Jacky, there was a moment
where her distress lifted into the air like a small puff of
acrid smoke, and the rest of the audience made a tiny
collective sigh as they detected it. Maarike went on. 'I
know his family think this is my fault, that I made a

wrong decision, and despite I know it woss a good decision – it just turned out wrong – I feel sad.'

Decisions about stopping medicines require bravery, and not just for doctors. We all weigh up the information and choose one option or another, and none of us knows what the future holds. Maarike's patient Jacky may easily have had that stroke anyway – blood thinners don't abolish risk; they just reduce it. Or he may have stayed on the blood thinner, and had more nose bleeds and trips to hospital, and have become exhausted and succumbed to an infection. Doctors get used to making decisions, and must learn to accept outcomes that aren't what we hoped for. But the move to shared decision-making, to Mangin's team's approach to polypharmacy, where the patient is part of the team – well, that extends responsibility to patients themselves, or to families, friends or carers making decisions on their behalf. For many people that feels a big burden. Even when my patient has been given good information he may feel anxious that he will make the wrong decision, and that feeling tends to be even more intense when we are making such decisions on behalf of someone we love. Thus these decisions can demand a certain pinch of courage. We all – doctors, patients, families or carers – need to be able to feel that we have come to a conclusion in good faith. We must trust not only the information we are given but our own judgement, and we must be prepared not to feel bad about what happens next. Good decisions can turn out wrong.

Peggy, Joe and I turned to the third pile of medicines. By the time she left clinic she would be taking tablets that either made her feel better, or that she felt sure were doing her good. She would have stopped taking those doing harm, and those that were not working, and we would have made some decisions together about which of the preventive medicines she would like to continue. Peggy might still rattle, but less, and with more confidence.

*

A good place to find more information about drugs and the likelihood of their helping is here:
   http://www.polypharmacy.scot.nhs.uk/polypharmacy-guidance-medicines-review/

One of several studies linking anticholinergic drugs with dementia is here:
   https://www.bmj.com/content/361/bmj.k1315

A representative study of medication-related harm in frailty is here:
   https://academic.oup.com/ageing/article/48/Supplement _1/i27/5308747

UK data about the incidence of multiple chronic conditions with age is here:

https://www.ageuk.org.uk/Documents/EN-GB/For-
professionals/Research/Age_UK_almanac_FINAL_9
Oct15.pdf?dtrk=true

You can watch Dr Dee Mangin talking about the TAPER
deprescribing project here:
https://taper.fammedmcmaster.ca/

And her team's paper about patient and carer views is
here:
https://www.ncbi.nlm.nih.gov/pmc/articles/PMC645
2573/

Here is the terrific paper Mangin wrote in 2007 with Iona
Heath and Kieran Sweeney about preventive medicines
in old age:
https://www.ncbi.nlm.nih.gov/pmc/articles/PMC194
1858/

8. Choosing Wisely

Doxycycline is a marvellous drug. It has anti-inflammatory properties that makes it useful for some nasty skin conditions, and it's effective for the prevention of malaria in many parts of the world; it's a widely used antibiotic, and is cheap as chips. I put together a medicine chest for my husband to take on a tropical surfing trip and included a box of doxycycline, writing instructions on the carton, *For chest infections and pussy*, then running out of space, continuing with *wounds* on the back, meaning wounds with pus. He was delighted. Anyway, doxycycline is very handy, and you only have to take it once a day, and I was not worried when I was prescribed it for an annoying rash around my eyes, even when I was warned I'd need a two-month course. But doxycycline can make you feel sick, and it did that to me, so I sensibly took it at night, before going to bed, in order that I could sleep through the nausea. In due course I started getting a very saddening pain in my chest, which got worse, until I thought something essential might be tearing inside, and I took myself to the Emergency Department, where whirling, smiling staff checked my heart, but the next day even swallowing water brought tears to my eyes, and one of the kind gastroenterologists looked down my throat with an endoscope ('We can do it with or without sedation, patient's choice. You're having sedation.') and found that I'd developed a big raw ulcer in my oesophagus, and my dear colleague Bella brandished the doxycycline information leaflet at me, saying, 'Luce, you idiot,' and showing me where it warns, *You should take the capsules well before you go to bed for the night to stop ulceration of your gullet. It is important not to lie down for at least thirty minutes after taking doxycycline capsules.* It was all very embarrassing.

In a report in 2012 the World Health Organization (WHO) estimated that globally 'more than half of all medicines are prescribed, dispensed or sold inappropriately', and went on to explain that the 'overuse, underuse or misuse of medicines results in wastage of scarce resources and widespread health hazards'. I've spent much of the last chapter complaining about how difficult prescribing is for doctors. But try being a patient! I only had to take one tablet and I got that wrong. My patients, the patients of geriatricians, face much bigger problems. Medicines that you must take before, after or with a meal; while standing or sitting; only on a Tuesday; not before driving; not at the same time as any of the others; not with alcohol or milk or grapefruit juice or broccoli or Brussels sprouts. Medicines that must be chewed or crushed or dissolved, but only in water or apple puree, or must instead be swallowed whole but are the size of a horse pill, and you wonder whether rather than swallowing them you wouldn't be better off inserting them at the other end. Medicines that each have an alias, a trade name in big print and a generic one in small print; medicines that aren't the same as last week's, or maybe they are, but the packaging, shape and colour have all changed. Or they look like the same medicine, but when you peer closely they are a different dose. Medicines that look pretty but don't work, like docusate, probably the world's most useless laxative. And you must take medicines that the local pharmacy usually has in stock but hasn't got today, and you must come back tomorrow for the one they don't have, but they've given you more of the ones you have a pile of already. Medicines, one of which might be giving you that metallic taste or making you feel dizzy or just uneasy but it's hard to say which one it is. And perhaps you might be like my patient Heinrich, finding the instructions so fussy that it's easier if you pop them all out of their packets and into an empty tissue box, and choose seven of the dolly mixtures to take each day; or like Iris you might even have a secret mountain of plastic drug-dispensing trays in the kitchen cupboard, and you might have opened a few of the foil-covered compartments, but have left many untouched, and the trays look like sad Advent calendars with random doors torn open.

There's a growing international realization that more is not necessarily better, that any healthcare interventions – scans, blood tests, cancer treatments, surgical procedures, as well as daily medicines – can bring harm as well as benefit. In Scotland, country of cool-headed rationality, a campaign was launched in 2016 called Realistic Medicine, demanding that we become better at 'having or showing a sensible and practical idea of what can be achieved or expected', as well as 'representing things in a way that is accurate and true to life'. The Realistic Medicine team requires that those providing care 'have the courage to be honest, open and balanced'.

A global campaign, Choosing Wisely, encourages conversations that allow patients' views to be heard. Phrases like 'no decision about me, without me' now ring out, part of a worldwide mission to amplify the patient's voice, and the Choosing Wisely group suggests that people facing any kind of treatment decision could try BRAN, and ask what are the Benefits? What are the Risks? What are the Alternatives? And what happens if I do Nothing?

I made such a mess of my own treatment. Why didn't I even read the leaflet? The first reason, and not one that usually applies to my patients, was arrogance. I thought I knew everything about doxycycline. And perhaps I thought too that the doctor prescribing it would warn me of side effects, so it wasn't my job to read the instructions. And, most importantly, I just wasn't very interested. I wanted my rash to go away, and that was all.

The WHO reported again on misuse of medications and other treatments in 2017, launching an initiative called Global Patient Safety. The authors wrote: *Patients and the public . . . are too often made to be passive recipients of medicines and not informed and empowered to play their part in making the process of medication safer.*

I was not made to be a passive recipient. I chose that role. But many people *are* made to feel that they don't have a say. Sometimes we are made passive because we are told our doctor is busy, and we don't want to take his time. Or perhaps we like him and don't want to upset him by saying we don't trust or take the tablets. Perhaps we feel a little afraid of our doctor, and we worry that she will be angry. Sometimes we feel we don't have 'our' doctor at all, and it'll be a different one again, and we'll have to start the whole story at the beginning. Sometimes we feel guilty – we feel we have a duty to take the medicines, or to have the test, that we have a duty to stay well, and we worry that these tablets or tests are all that stand between us and a bad thing happening. Or we may be forgetful and keep quiet, because we're sure someone explained these tablets but we can't quite remember what they said. Sometimes the explanation is just too complicated – we feel we'd need a PhD in pharmacology to understand the options. Sometimes we're not convinced that the person doing the explaining – the pharmacist, the GP, the nurse or the hospital specialist – really grasps our situation and understands what we want to get from the care that's on offer.

So how can we best strengthen our hand, abandon passivity and become an active participant? The honesty and openness demanded by the Realistic Medicine campaign seems to work both ways. I could have taken more responsibility for my treatment. I spend my life reminding students and young doctors of the hazards of medicines, and completely failed to follow the basic instructions to keep myself safe. What demands can we make of ourselves as patients?

It is reasonable to have an idea what each of our medications is for. If we don't know, we must ask. And if it should be alleviating some specific symptom, and doesn't seem to be working, we must say so.

It is reasonable to read the instructions and the side-effect list and to consider whether we are being detrimentally affected – and if we are, again, we must say so. I listened to Eileen's signature cough at our village events for years – a little 'ahem' – before one day she showed me her tablets, among which was ramipril, a blood pressure tablet that, like all drugs in its family (their name ends with 'pril'), gives about one in ten people a dry cough. And it turned out Eileen knew that, but didn't like to mention it to her doctor, feeling she should not make a fuss, and so did not know that there's a good alternative that doesn't cause coughs, and she had eight years or so of broken sleep that didn't need to happen, and that may even have offset any benefit the reduction in her blood pressure was bringing.

We must not get bogged down in worrying about rare side effects, but it's reasonable to inform ourselves at least about the common ones: for example, that all painkillers stronger than paracetamol, those in the opioid class, which includes codeine and tramadol, and things like fentanyl patches (which look like nothing at all, innocuous sticking plasters, but are extremely potent) – that all these will cause constipation in almost everyone, and that constipation may be severe, and will almost always require a decent laxative from the start, not just an extra prune or two and waiting to see if it gets better. These drugs will also cause drowsiness and confusion in many, especially those who are frail and already drowsy or confused. And rare side effects do happen, so if we develop some new symptom, it's sensible to read the small print and make the connection between what we are taking and how we are feeling.

It's reasonable if we are taking any long-term medicine at all, to expect a review roughly annually of its benefits and risks. It's reasonable to ask, if we are offered something new, the BRAN questions. We must know the benefits, the risks and the alternatives, and what happens if we do nothing.

The medical students are playing a game; they've been given five cartons of medicines and I ask them to sort the drugs into the order in which they were prescribed. The boxes contain oxybutynin, amlodipine, ibuprofen, furosemide and eye drops. I add a big jar of senna. The students look worried and point out that there are no dates on the cartons.

'That doesn't matter – I want you to think about *why*

each drug was prescribed. Mrs Brooks was eighty-seven, and she went to see her doctor because of pain in her knee. A year later she was taking all of these.'

The students cotton on. They reach for the carton of ibuprofen, an anti-inflammatory drug, good for the arthritic pain in Mrs Brooks' knee. We talk about its potential side effects, and remember that although it's a useful painkiller and might be exactly what Mrs Brooks needed it can push blood pressure slightly upwards. One of the students puts the carton of amlodipine next in line; it's a drug to bring Mrs Brooks' blood pressure back down. Her colleague smiles as she realizes what happened next.

'Amlodipine can cause ankle swelling!' she says, and places the box of water tablets, furosemide, alongside the amlodipine.

'Exactly, you've got it,' I tell them. 'About one in ten people get ankle swelling on drugs in the amlodipine class. What happens when someone who is fifty gets swollen ankles on a blood pressure tablet?'

'They go back to their GP,' the students offer, 'and stop taking it.'

'That's true, and they'll be switched to a different blood pressure tablet, but when an older person has the same problem, swollen ankles, they get put on a water tablet, because . . .?'

'Because the doctor thinks they've got heart failure!'

Side effects happen more often in older people than in the young, but are also regarded differently in older people who tend to have other things wrong with them. It's easy to make a mistake; sometimes doctors don't realize that the bad thing happening is a side effect and think instead that it's a new condition.

'Just that. So now we have the ibuprofen pushing Mrs B's blood pressure up, the amlodipine to bring it back down, and the furosemide to treat the ankle swelling caused by the amlodipine. What happened next?'

The students haven't encountered oxybutinin before. I explain that it's another of the tablets designed to calm an overactive bladder. Poor Mrs Brooks, until she started taking the furosemide she could just about hold on until she reached a loo, but now her waterworks had begun an impatient campaign of disobedience. So she was given oxybutinin. And more side effects. What would they be?

The first student narrows her eyes as she remembers her pharmacology lectures. 'Oxybutinin must be an anticholinergic, is that right? So the side effects would be dry eyes, dry mouth, constipation . . .' She triumphantly places the artificial tears and the senna jar at the end of the line.

This is the prescribing cascade, each drug added to counter the side effects of another. Sometimes this is inescapable – the opioid painkillers call for a side order of laxatives. In certain situations pills contain the antidote for their own side effects; the essential medication for many people with Parkinson's disease, levodopa, would cause terrible vomiting if it were not cleverly combined in one pill with another drug that prevents the levodopa from affecting the stomach, targeting it instead to the brain where it's needed. So 'one drug for the side effect of another' may be vital, but often that's not the case, and rather than simply reaching for a second medication doctors and patients ought to step back and have a think about whether the benefit of the offending tablet is worth the price of its side effects. And benefit becomes harder to pin down when we're thinking about a medicine that isn't to treat existing symptoms, that doesn't make us feel better today, but is to change the risk of a future problem. How then can a patient make an active, informed decision?

Alongside that Realistic Medicine campaign, Scotland is tackling medications. The first step of Scotland's polypharmacy team is to ask each patient 'What matters to you?' Knowing what you want to get out of your treatments, being honest and open about it, helps decisions fall into place, and once all the right information is laid out in a way that makes sense many of these decisions are not as difficult for patients and families as they might look.

Charles was in clinic, wondering whether he should start taking a blood-thinning tablet. He was seventy-seven, and a few weeks previously his left arm had become suddenly weak while he was shopping. The cashier at the supermarket had noticed his face droop and her manager had called an ambulance, but within minutes of his arrival in ED Charles was back to rights.

He'd had a transient ischaemic attack (TIA), a 'mini-stroke'.

'They didn't find anything on the scans,' Charles told me, 'just the irregular heart rhythm on the heart recording.'

Charles, like Maarike's patient Jacky, had atrial fibrillation, which is the commonest of the electrical upsets to which the ageing heart is prone. Instead of beating regularly the upper chambers of his heart, his atria, were quivering with uncoordinated activity, while the important lower chambers got on with pumping blood around his lungs and body. AF often doesn't much affect the function of the heart pump – blood still goes round – but the flow of blood through the heart itself becomes uneven, and stagnant back eddies develop, and in these eddies small blood clots can form, which cause no harm while they stay where they are but may be carried out of the heart along the big blood vessels and into the brain, lodging there in some smaller but vital cerebral artery to produce a devastating stroke.

I explained this to Charles and continued. 'Being in AF, and having had a stroke, even a mini one, means you're at a higher risk of having another stroke. Taking a blood thinner, a proper anticoagulant rather than just aspirin, reduces that risk by about sixty per cent.'

'And the downside?' he asked.

'Well, being on an anticoagulant makes you more likely to bleed, which includes serious bleeding, not just bruises: a bleed into the brain, or into the stomach or gut.'

Charles pulled a face, and looked at his sock, exposed where his legs were crossed at the ankle. A green sock with reindeer.

'How do the numbers stack up?'

'I can show you.' I clicked the letters *CHADSVASC* into the computer to find a scoring system that would give us some hard figures about the chances of Charles having a stroke. I warned him as we waited for the screen to come up. 'Officially you'll be at high risk, even though you haven't got other factors.'

'My GP said that,' Charles agreed gloomily.

His past medical history was unblemished. We ticked no to questions about diabetes, high blood pressure, heart attacks. The computer calculated Charles's CHA_2DS_2-VASc score as four, and the web page announced that he was indeed at high risk of stroke.

Charles leaned past me to peer at the screen, and scrunched up his face as he read it to me. 'OK, so I score four, which it says here happens to give me an annual risk of stroke of four per cent. I don't call that high! That's a ninety-six per cent chance of *not* having a stroke this year. I've been waiting for the sky to fall on my head for nothing.'

Charles was right about what is high and what isn't. He had been given the impression that he was almost bound to have another stroke, imminently at that. To him a 4% annual risk seemed reassuringly low. To someone else a 4% chance – one in twenty-five – might feel frighteningly likely.

When I talked with Emily, who had the same risk score as Charles, I laid out the numbers for her on a piece of paper. A 4% chance of a stroke each year, which will come down to a bit under 2% on a blood thinner – but with an increased risk of bleeding. Somewhere between about 3 and 5% of people taking an anticoagulant will have a severe bleed each year. Emily barely glanced at the numbers, and straightened her shoulders firmly.

'My mother had a stroke. It was awful – it would have been better if she'd died really, but she didn't, and it was very hard for her.'

'High' to one person is not 'high' to another. So when we are told that something is 'high risk' or 'low probability', it is reasonable to ask what that really means. Doctors often can't be precise, but we should be able to give an impression of the scale of risk.

As a patient, once we have a feel for the likelihood of good or harm delivered by a treatment we can apply our own view. Some people who use the BRAN acronym create the word BRAIN instead, adding an 'I' to the list, which stands for 'Instinct'.

It is this extra dimension, the 'I', that helps make these decisions easier, and explains why we don't all make the same decisions. It's not 'instinct' in the sense of being able to guess what might be going to happen to us next, or having some strange intuition that we're better off one way or another; rather, it's our knowledge of what's gone before and what we hope for next, our own experience, that makes the path clear. And that's also why as a doctor I can't make these decisions for you. I can answer the BRAN questions: for Charles, data and guidelines suggested he would have a lower risk of stroke and even death if he started a blood thinner, but it was Charles who knew that he disliked pills and had a lifelong aversion to blood, and would decline the anti-coagulant; and Emily conversely knew she would do anything, would accept almost any odds, to reduce her risk of having a stroke. Perhaps we could call that 'I', not instinct, but 'Individuality' instead. Charles's wife backed his decision, telling me, 'He's not really a pill person. He's more of a water-divining, Buddhism and homeopathy sort.'

What else can make treatment decisions less difficult? It helps, I think, to remember that for many older people who are also frail, the benefits and burdens of many treatments are uncertain, and may often be close to equipoise. We are given the impression that all the medicines are essential (that happens particularly to families looking after someone who has dementia), but often that isn't true.

I must be fearsomely clear here: you should not simply stop a medicine (for yourself or anyone else) without talking to a professional who knows you and your medical history. But you are entitled to have that conversation.

There are a few medicines that are preventing some dire and immediate calamity, like certain epilepsy medicines for people who really do have epilepsy, or insulin for the truly insulin-dependent diabetic (insulin started in later life, for better control of the type 2 diabetes usually treated by tablets, is a different matter). Many medications can be stopped without something dramatic happening, others need to be weaned down gradually, but few are truly essential, and knowing this may help relieve some of the anxiety that accompanies these conversations.

Towards the end, for people who may be in their last year of life, or for those who have severe dementia, treatments need to be scrutinized even more carefully. The chance that they are helping becomes smaller and their burden becomes heavier, not just through potential side effects, but the sheer effort of taking them. The goal of treatment may have changed. It can be hard to be honest and open. We might wonder if it is OK to say, 'My husband has terrible dementia. He would not wish to live this way. Can we talk about stopping the medicines that are not making him better but are meant to be keeping him alive?' *Of course* it is OK to say this. It is not a bad thing to say. In fact, it may be the best thing to say.

At another training day one of the most experienced GPs put his hand up. I like and admire him and was taken aback to find him aggrieved.

'Right, Lucy, are there any drugs you *do* actually like?'

There are few things more joyous than watching someone with newly diagnosed Parkinson's disease becoming unlocked by a supply of dopamine. Getting a driving licence back, for someone whose epilepsy is now controlled. Seeing the grating agony of a gouty joint subside after a smidgen of colchicine. Finding the night's icy-nosed, frightened patient with decompensated heart failure tucking into the morning's tea and toast after an emergency dose of diuretics. Observing the clarity, the relief, when an infection-related delirium has been banished by judicious antibiotics. And no self-respecting geriatrician would approach a desert island without good laxatives.

Many drugs, operations and other treatments make an important positive difference to people's lives. But treatments can also cause harm. Doctors have always tended to overestimate benefit and underestimate harm – this has been proven in multiple studies – and we know less than we should about whether a treatment will work in very old people, especially in those who have frailty. We need to apply good knowledge where it exists, but also must be honest.

There is a final thread hanging loose when we talk about treatment decisions with very old people and their families. I bumped into Lisa, whose children went to playgroup with mine years ago. These days her father lives with the family and had recently returned home after a spell in hospital. Lisa was not pleased.

'They just stopped half his medicines. I don't know

why, and Dad hasn't a clue.' She frowned. 'I know he was on a lot, but he must've been on them for a reason.'

And I can guess that Lisa worried that her dad's treatments had been stopped because he is old, because the NHS is broke, because he's not worth it. And it is true that healthcare is constrained, that NICE deliberates over expensive drugs and treatments and withholds approval when the cost is too high. I like Scotland's polypharmacy campaign, with its clear advice for patients and professionals, but it contains a tiny disingenuous component. The information for patients talks about a process of several steps to getting medicines right – working out what matters, thinking about side effects and talking about whether the medicines are working and other good things, but the information for professionals includes one more step, which is not in the patient information, and that is a consideration of cost. And the fact that this appears in one part of the guidance, but not in the part for patients, makes me uneasy, because it suggests that there is something to cover up here when there isn't.

Older people, even very old people, are entitled to and are given heroic treatment when this stands a sensible chance of success and is what they want. And the Scottish polypharmacy team's advice is clear, saying, 'Changing drugs for cost reasons should only be considered if effectiveness, safety or adherence would not be compromised.'

Everyone would agree that it is wrong – unethical

even – to offer a treatment that does not work or is unwanted or is unnecessarily expensive; and because most drugs can be sourced from a variety of manufacturers at different costs it's wise for prescribers to shop around. We should be as open and honest about that process as everything else. Getting medicines and treatments perfect is not about NHS penny-pinching, and 'rational' prescribing is not the same as 'rationed' prescribing, but without proper discussion and explanation this is how it can seem. Lisa's dad's drugs may well have been doing him no good, or even harming him, but changing them should have been discussed with him or with Lisa on his behalf, because otherwise they are both left feeling that his health, his life, is of limited worth, and that is not right.

I'm having a cup of tea with Ron and Stella in their kitchen where a wall calendar shows photographs of hefty and contented-looking cows. Ron has reiterated with spicy vigour his views on the Environment Agency, and the state of the rhynes, the great drainage channels that run across this low-lying land. Now Stella is talking, and Ron has stood up and is leaning uneasily on the table, moving from side to side and wincing, and Stella stops to look at her husband with concern, and I ask, 'What did they say about the foot?' For I know Ron's foot and how its structure has collapsed, and how his weight now lands on what was once its arch, and how his heel has turned so that his inner ankle bone brushes the floor, and the skin is stretched tight and shiny and red. And I know that he's tried painkillers and braces, and a special boot was made for him that doesn't fit, and that Ron pushes his foot back into his old boot and laces it up, so that he can go down the garden to look at the barn where his cattle once steamed in the frost, and to attend to cauliflowers that must be carried in both arms. I know that Ron has had an appointment with an orthopaedic surgeon, a foot and ankle specialist, to consider an operation, and now Ron shakes his head and sets his hand on the table, implacable. Fingers spread wide.

'No. Too busted. Too old. Not worth it.'

And I nod and we move on to talk about Ron's wooden whistle that he deploys surreptitiously in early spring to make the sound of the first cuckoo, but afterwards I think about Ron's words, and hope that he knows where the lack of worth lies. Because that operation, a triple arthrodesis to reshape and fuse together the bones of his foot, is a big one, and would involve a hospital stay, screws and pins and strong painkillers, and then several weeks of being barred from putting any weight at all through the leg, which means hopping on his opposite hip, which is also crumbling, and many more weeks of being in a cast, and a considerable risk of infection or of the wound breaking or of the bones failing to knit back together, so there's no guarantee of his pain being eventually relieved, and Ron's situation may be made worse rather than better. His orthopaedic surgeon has thought about Ron's dicky heart and his other medical problems, and has been honest and open, as requested by those empowering campaigns, about the chances of successful surgery. So, my friend Ron, the lack of worth lies in the treatment, not in the patient.

I often look at a tablet, and think, *That medicine is* not good enough *for my patient. It doesn't work well enough; it's not making things better enough.* It is the treatment that is not good enough for the patient, rather than the patient who is not good enough for the treatment. It is the operation that is not worth it. You, Ron, are worth everything.

9. 'We Didn't Like to Say It'

Margaret Whitmore looks worried. She was admitted to hospital last night and is now sitting in the chair beside her bed, her toast is untouched, and her gaze darts around the ward as she tries to make sense of her surroundings. A white hanky with an embroidered flower is held tightly in her left fist, and her right hand plays around with the top button of her nightdress.

We've read through Margaret's notes and results already – the admission slip says *worsening confusion*, and the team downstairs have made a diagnosis of urinary infection. This is frequently a wrong diagnosis, and it's important to check that something else isn't missed, but urinary tract infections, UTIs, are very common, and often make older people muddled. This time Margaret's blood results, tender tummy and high temperature suggest that the team's on the right track.

Today my registrar Sarah is taking my place on the ward round, and I'm observing her work. Sarah introduces herself, and me, and points out our youngest doctor, Cerys. Margaret glances warily at me before looking back at Sarah as she hunkers down beside the chair.

'I'm sorry you've landed up in hospital,' says Sarah. 'You must be feeling all shaken up.'

Margaret tips her head to one side, but doesn't say anything.

Sarah goes on. 'Mrs Whitmore, I know this sounds like a silly question –' Margaret gives a little smile – 'but do you know where you are? Can you tell me the name of this place?'

'Yes,' says Margaret, suddenly confident. 'It's . . . it's . . .'

She looks around again, then down at her hand, defeated.

Sarah rescues her deftly. 'Don't worry, it's hard to keep track of things in here. You've not been well, and you're in hospital –' she names it – 'and we think you've got an infection and you're going to get better.'

Margaret bows her head and puts her hand in front of her eyes, rubbing her forehead as she tries to take in this information. Sarah is reassuring and gentle – she makes sure that Margaret's not in pain, examines her for signs of infection elsewhere, looks at the drug chart carefully to be certain there's nothing on it that might be making things worse, and checks that a suitable antibiotic has been chosen. She has a chat with Margaret's nurse, Raul, who is aware that Margaret is at high risk of having a fall – she tried to get up this morning without help and was very wobbly. Raul's made sure she's been given one of the most visible beds on the ward. He and Jackie, the healthcare assistant, are checking often whether she needs anything or wants to go to the bathroom.

We write Margaret's problem list. Number one is easy – UTI – but then we are stuck. Margaret is confused, but how normal is this for her? Sarah, Cerys and I talk about the need for a collateral history – we need to hear from someone who knows Margaret and can tell us what she's usually like.

Later that morning, we are seeing another patient when Cerys notices that Margaret's family are visiting.

'Could you have a chat with them,' I ask Cerys, 'and see how she usually is?'

Cerys is back in a few minutes and reports, 'She's not usually confused. That's her husband and daughter, and they say she's fine at home.'

Lots of things can make people become suddenly very confused, a condition called delirium. It can happen to anyone, the brain getting derailed from its normal thinking processes. Sometimes delirium causes agitation; more commonly, and easier to miss, delirium can make people quiet, withdrawn or sleepy. The man with malaria, silently slipping in and out of consciousness in a tropical hospital, is delirious, and the lad outside the nightclub in a state of intoxicated agitation has a form of delirium.

In older people less dramatic provocations are enough to set things awry. The ageing brain, like other parts of the body, has less reserve; it's vulnerable. This vulnerable brain is less able to cope with challenges like infections and drugs and variations in the levels of various chemicals in the blood, such as sugar or sodium or thyroid hormones. When I'm teaching medical students we talk about more subtle things that might contribute.

I ask them to think of things that would affect themselves, which would prevent them from concentrating while trying to complete an exam paper; they suggest having slept badly; a hangover from taking a sleeping tablet; too much noise; an uncomfortable chair; or needing a pee. I agree – all these can also make older people more confused, as can being worried, depressed, bereaved or in pain. As a brave woman explained to me, describing how confused she had been when she broke her arm, 'I was so *distracted* by the pain, I couldn't think straight. I couldn't answer the simplest question.' Delirium can develop quickly, even in those whose brain has been working well, and it happens more easily in those who already have a brain problem such as dementia. Simple constipation can provoke delirium in someone vulnerable, and delirium's often due to a combination of several apparently small things. Admission to hospital with its bright lights, strange smells and bewildering array of faces, may derail yet further someone's ability to think.

We update Margaret's problem list. *1. UTI 2. Delirium.*

Sarah asks Cerys, 'Do you think Margaret might have dementia too?'

'Oh, I'm not sure. Her family said she's not like this at home. They think she's usually OK.'

We take Margaret's family to the little sitting room behind the nurses' station, and her husband Brian tells Sarah how bad she's been in the last few days, getting dressed in the middle of the night ready to go shopping; how he's found her lost in the bathroom, unable to find

her way back to bed. She has been going through cupboards, trying to find food for the cat, which died last
year, and she's torn a magazine page into shreds.

'She's not like this,' Brian says, and his hand shakes a
little on his walking stick, his cuff loose at his wrist. 'She
was all right, back along.'

Sarah explains that we think Margaret's got a urine
infection and that we hope she'll get better once the
antibiotic starts working.

'Mr Whitmore, I was wondering, before she got this
infection, is Margaret's memory usually as sharp as it
used to be?'

Brian frowns slightly and tips his head from side to
side in a 'yes and no' movement.

Sarah goes on. 'Who does the shopping and the cooking at home?'

'We do it together. She peels the veg. She can get a bit
mixed up with the oven now.'

'What about the shopping list?'

'Oh, I do that. She likes to add a few bits but I've got
a routine.'

'And are you the driver?'

'I am indeed. Mr Taxi-man. She gave up the driving a
couple of years back.'

'Why was that?'

Brian looks uncomfortable, and his daughter Christine joins in. 'Mum got in a muddle down in Sidmouth.
It was really busy and she lost us and couldn't find the
car . . .'

'It sounds as if you're doing a great job driving her, Mr Whitmore,' Sarah says. 'What about the bills, and getting things mended around the house?'

'Oh, she wouldn't be able to do that.' Brian shakes his head firmly. 'She used to, but these days she'd get worried. I've done them the last few years. And she doesn't like using the new phone either.'

Sarah continues her exploration. There are good things. Margaret is always happy to see the grandchildren. She takes care of her appearance and dresses neatly each day. She eats well. She doesn't go out alone for fear of getting lost, but she and Brian go to church every week, which she enjoys, and on Tuesdays they go skittling with friends – Margaret doesn't play, but she likes the chat. She can tell the family about her childhood in Essex, but she wouldn't remember her daughter's birthday now, and tends to mistake one grandchild for another. Christine tells us, 'Mum's memory's not great. But it's fine. She's not confused, not like this.'

'She's doing well.' Sarah puts her hand on Brian's. 'And you're doing a great job. But I think her memory problems are a bit more than just what happens when you get older.'

We are again in that familiar situation, as with falls, of working out what is 'common but not normal'. Margaret's memory loss is more significant than the simple forgetfulness of ageing. And her problems at home, before this recent illness, are with more than memory alone. Her everyday life has been affected, with Brian taking on many of her roles, his quiet assumption of responsibility masking the disintegration of Margaret's mind.

Sarah treads carefully, pausing before saying, 'I'm afraid I think Margaret probably has dementia. Does that sound possible to you?'

Brian and his daughter exchange looks.

Christine says, 'We thought it might be that, didn't we, Dad? But we didn't like to say it.'

Oh, the big D, dementia, and how much we don't like to say it. It's a word primed with emotion, pinned in the thoughts of many to images of loss, fear, indignity. It's politically charged too, because of the colossal mess of funding (or lack of it) for social care. Alongside that dementia has somehow been monetized; looking for statistics on the internet, you are hit with listings for 'the dementia industry' and 'dementia global market reports'. And dementia has become an arena for philosophical scrapping, between those who focus relentlessly on the positive, who will not allow 'Gerry has dementia' but instead insist upon 'Gerry is living with dementia', and an opposing team, who dwell on the negatives, the shortcomings of certain care homes, the obliteration of personality. And in between the two camps, somewhere between music and ice cream and loneliness and continence pads, hundreds of thousands of people with dementia and their families are getting on with life, muddling along and doing their best.

*

Before we had children various of our friends had infants who were picky eaters, and I would feel privately aggrieved that these parents hadn't addressed the problem, hadn't applied properly the advice of myriad guides to toddler taming, or of TV super-nannies or their own mothers. Surely these competent adults should not be held to ransom by an infuriating three-year-old implacably picking the raisins out of her garibaldi biscuit? And then we had our son, who at eighteen months abruptly closed his mouth to breakfast cereal, potatoes, peas, jam, chicken and almost every other foodstuff, and for two years he ate only bread and butter, and we were given a great deal of advice, and absolutely nothing worked.

I am wary then of presenting suggestions that may be irritating, patronizing or simply wrong for the situation, not applicable to someone's father, wife or partner. There's a saying that 'when you have met someone who has dementia you have met someone who has dementia', and it is important to pay more than lip service to the fact that everyone is individual, and their relationships are unique. In addition, although I've been involved in the care of many people with dementia – several thousand, I guess – and have helped my own family members with dementia, I have not lived the experience: of being given a dementia diagnosis or living in the same house, the same room, as someone who has dementia, day in, day out, for years and years. So the rest of this chapter and the next, and any other mention of the care of those who have dementia, is offered with some hesitation, and with considerable respect.

This book isn't a comprehensive guide to life with dementia. There are great resources available and you've only got to stick the word into a search engine to find good advice – the NHS Choices website, and the Alzheimer's Society one, are informative, clear and kind. Information is available in hospitals and GP surgeries, and there will be details there too of local sources of help. There are sympathetic books written by thoughtful, experienced people.

It might be helpful, however, if I describe some of the conversations regarding dementia that patients and families have with geriatricians (and psychogeriatricians, doctors with a training in psychiatry rather than internal medicine; our work overlaps in some areas, and psychogeriatricians care for very many people with dementia, especially those who do not have concurrent physical illnesses). Notwithstanding the towering importance of individual experience, patterns emerge, and there are problems, misperceptions and questions that are held in common. The areas where I perhaps see most unhappiness, and where good information can make a positive difference, come under two broad themes: one is the path to the diagnosis of dementia, and the other is how we respond to that diagnosis.

Each of those themes delivers a slew of questions, some easy to ask, others held in our hearts: secret questions. How do you know if someone's got dementia? Is there a scan? Why bother finding out if there's so little you can do about it anyway? And then: what am I supposed to actually *do* now that you've told me I have dementia? What are we to expect? The unspoken questions: should my husband keep taking all these medicines designed to prevent a heart attack when he's always said he wants to die suddenly, quickly, presumably therefore of a heart attack? Why are the doctors still treating Mum's infections when she is in such a terrible state? How may I continue to love someone whose behaviour is beyond my capacity for understanding and forgiveness?

Officially dementia isn't really an illness; the word describes a set of symptoms, and there are many different illnesses that cause dementia. Alzheimer's disease is the commonest of these. Vascular dementia comes next – a series of strokes, or just one bad stroke, that affect the parts of the brain involved in thinking, language and memory, rather than only the parts that control power and movement. Many people have both Alzheimer's and vascular dementia. Then there's dementia with Lewy bodies (DLB), worth knowing about because it has a special pattern. And there are other forms: frontotemporal dementia, which may come with particularly upsetting changes in behaviour, and the sort of dementia people get who have had Parkinson's disease for many years, and rarer sorts still.

What then are the symptoms of dementia? Many people are aware that dementia affects not just memory, but also other areas of thinking, like organizational skills, planning, orientation, language. But perhaps it's not so obvious that dementia may affect other more nebulous, less measurable aspects of thought. There may be a sad erosion of curiosity, or of humour; of the appreciation of beauty; of the ability to empathize and to take an interest in others – in short a wearing thin of the characteristics that help us to be kind, interesting, likeable or even lovable.

How do you know if someone's got dementia? How do I know if *I* have got dementia? When I ask the students to tell me what questions they would ask of a family like Margaret's, they often start, 'Has she forgotten her husband's name? Does she remember to eat? Can she get dressed properly, and get to the toilet?' But these questions are not discerning; Margaret doesn't have any of those difficulties. What about earlier, subtler signs of trouble?

I ask the students to think about children. By the time they get to primary school most small children have learned to use a knife and fork, and can dress themselves and use the loo. Most people hang on to these basic abilities for a long while; these 'primary-school skills' are lost late. I ask the students to tell me instead what teenagers are learning. What are my own dear children, between fifteen and twenty-one, now getting the hang of? Phoning their friends and planning a social life. Driving and using public transport in strange cities. Deploying a richer, more elaborate vocabulary. Planning meals and cooking. Keeping their rooms clean and tidy (up to a point – it's a role-model problem). Finding somewhere to live and a job, and managing their finances. Travelling, and telling us their stories when they return without repeating themselves.

The students can now see what skills may be lost earliest by those who are developing dementia. People who have learned several languages tend to lose them in reverse order; I watched my stalwart patient Ilse gradually lose the English vocabulary she had used confidently for decades, slipping back to the German of her childhood. Friendships become untended, and families help set up direct debits and start checking through the post for unpaid bills without thinking much about it. Mum takes ages to work out how to use the new microwave, or Dad tells us again about his problem getting the local garage to fix the car. Long-term memory may be preserved, but what happened at lunchtime today is lost. Personalities may change, subtly at first – the placid may become anxious, or the irritable may develop a sunny outlook. My friend Siân says, 'Dad was called Grumpy Grandpa for good reason, but now he's all smiles. I think he's forgotten everything he used to worry about.'

How else can we tell if someone has dementia? Memory tests aren't infallible. It's not fair to test someone's memory when they may be recovering from delirium, such as when they're getting over an infection or have been taking opiate medicines like codeine for pain.

Also, performance on memory tests can fluctuate, and sometimes those with a borderline score do better another day, and in any case dementia is not defined by memory alone. And people with a high educational level often score well on memory tests, even when their family know that they are in real trouble with everyday decisions.

I watched in admiration as Gilbert, a retired civil servant, dealt with his memory assessment. His worsening domestic chaos and increasingly haphazard social arrangements were worrying his friends, but he stormed through the 'recall' section of the test. Gilbert was asked to name as many animals as he could in one minute. Even people with no memory problems tend to run into trouble with this. Under pressure they might start off confidently: 'Dog, cat, cow,' then pause and veer off, slightly panicky, '. . . horse, pony – is both all right?' And they flounder a little before getting back on track: '. . . monkey, shark . . . umm . . . are fish allowed?'

Not Gilbert. 'Any animals, one minute?' Instructions confirmed, he set off. 'Right. Anteater. Badger. Coyote. Dolphin. Elephant. Faun.'

Gilbert was speeding up now, as he anchored his memory to the alphabet.

'Goat. Hippopotamus. Iguana. Jackal. Kangaroo. Llama. Manatee.'

A momentary hesitation – I suspected that he was savouring 'manatee' rather than struggling for the next word. He charged on: 'Newt, okapi, porpoise,' reaching 'zebra' with triumph. More detailed neuro-cognitive testing may have unmasked enough to produce a firm diagnosis – perhaps of frontotemporal dementia, given Gilbert's tendency to offer disparaging comments on their appearance, clothing or scent to his long-suffering helpers – but these assessments are scantily available outside research units, and Gilbert wasn't interested. No dementia diagnosis for him.

The path to a diagnosis is hard to find for other reasons. Sometimes it is camouflaged by symptoms that don't fit the standard template, which fool the eye and dupe us all.

Dilly was crocheting a square – intricate patterns of pale blue and green – when we reached her on the ward round.

'I make them for the new babies, you know, the early ones, what are they called?'

'Neonates?' I offered. 'Or premmies?'

'That's the ones, premmies,' said Dilly, and smoothed the square, her fingers passing over a sagging holey patch marring her otherwise regular stitches. I admired the pattern and asked whether Dilly had always been good at making things. 'Did it for my job,' she said brightly. 'Made new upholstery for old camper vans – cushions and curtains – enjoyed it.'

Dilly had been admitted a day ago, bewildered and drowsy. She'd been found outside her house, sitting on a wall, soaked through in the rain, but today she seemed on the ball. Like Margaret, she'd been diagnosed with a urine infection, but her blood tests were all normal and she didn't seem to have any symptoms apart from being muddled. Nothing on scans or X-rays, and even her urine sample had just been reported crystal clear. We scored the antibiotics off her chart and waited for her son to arrive.

Dave came in that afternoon by which time Dilly was asleep. I'd seen her earlier, tottering slightly as she made her way with small steps to the toilet, steadying herself at a bedside table as she passed.

'Mum, wake up, we're talking about you,' said Dave, a big chap with a burgundy polo shirt stretched over his comfortable girth.

Dilly shook herself and gave a couple of theatrical blinks, before sitting up to join the conversation.

'This is, what, the third, fourth, infection you've had this year, Mum?' said Dave, and Dilly agreed, saying, 'On and off antibiotics like a yo-yo.'

Dave went on. 'And you get in a right mix-up every time, all doolally, and you've fallen over I don't know how often, lots . . .'

'Not this time,' said Dilly defensively.

'No, but you're a perambulating jelly,' said Dave, and Dilly rolled her eyes.

'What's your memory like, Dilly?' I asked, and she laughed.

'Blimmin' awful. I don't know what's what half the time.'

I asked whether she had good days and bad days, and

now Dave rolled *his* eyes, and joined in. 'Definitely up and down, and on a good day, Mum, you're sharp as a tack, like when Rita came over, and then the next day you were away with the fairies and you got me mixed up with Michael.'

Dilly made that little raised eyebrow look that conveys 'I'm not sure I believe you, but I won't argue', and I asked her another thing.

'Dilly, I know this sounds an odd question, but are there times when your imagination plays tricks on you? Do you ever see something like a little dog or an animal and when you look again it isn't there?'

Dilly smiled, wrinkling her nose and saying, 'The little dog, he pops in and out,' and Dave looked surprised and said, 'You didn't tell me that, Mum!'

She replied, 'Well, I did say it to Michael, but he said it wasn't there, so I didn't go on about it. Anyhow, it's the little black dog, like the one we had in Kent.'

It was Dave's turn to pull a 'have it your own way' face now.

I asked Dilly, 'I wonder if there's sometimes people who aren't there either, like they're real but other people can't see them?'

She smiled serenely, telling us, 'Not very often, but sometimes they're in the corner; they're probably just the neighbours, but they're no trouble.'

Dilly's symptoms are classic of dementia with Lewy bodies. In 1910 Friedrich Lewy was a young scientist working in Berlin when he noticed tiny clumps of strange protein in some brain specimens. Lewy and others realized that these microscopic round balls were a common finding in the lower part of the brain, the brain stem, of people who had Parkinson's disease. The brain stem is concerned with movement, and with many of the 'automatic' functions of the nervous system, such as the control of blood pressure, sweating and the pupils of our eyes getting bigger in the dark; it doesn't do any conscious thinking or store memories. But many years later other pathologists discovered that in those with a particular pattern of behaviour, these strange protein clumps, now called Lewy bodies, could be found scattered all over the brain, affecting aspects of conscious thought in addition to giving the movement problems that are the hallmark of Parkinson's disease. People who have dementia with Lewy bodies often baffle their families, because their alertness and memory vary so much from day to day (and, later in the disease, even from hour to hour). Their children phone one another, saying, 'I just had the weirdest conversation with Dad,' but the next day it's as if nothing happened. It's common for people with DLB to be treated for infections that aren't there, because medical teams fear their patient may have delirium due to a urine or chest infection. People with DLB may also look as if they have Parkinson's disease – they may get stiff and shuffly, or develop a tremor and are prone to falling, but the levodopa tablets, so useful in Parkinson's disease, have a minimal or transient effect. And hallucinations are a famous feature of DLB, occurring much more often in this form of dementia than others. The hallucinations are often like Dilly's; they tend to be visual, and are 'vital and vivid' – not just smudgy shapes but living creatures, colourful and convincing, cats and rats and the man from the newsagent's, and while they can be frightening for some many others seem untroubled by these unexpected visitors, and decide not to mention them to family and friends.

Is there a scan for dementia? No, is the easy answer. We often do a scan, but it's mostly to look for other things that could cause memory problems. Scans can give a hint as to what *sort* of dementia someone has, but they aren't sensitive enough to tell whether someone has the illness. We might look at a CT scan in which the brain frankly looks like a walnut, shrunken and full of shaded areas indicating furred-up arteries and limited blood flow, yet find that our patient is contentedly completing day-to-day tasks without difficulty. Severe changes on a scan predict trouble ahead, but not for everyone. Equally many people with memory problems have scans that don't look bad; Margaret's scan, and Dilly's, were fine – not quite a twenty-year-old's, but not worrying either. So being told 'your scan looks normal' doesn't mean you have been given the all-clear for dementia. We can't see dementia on a scan.

So, is it worth getting a diagnosis? Would it be better just not to know?

First, many people who fear they may have dementia do not have dementia, and often we can provide reassurance that perceived problems lie within the bounds of 'normal'. My colleague Adam fielded the concerns of a meticulous wife nervous for her husband's brain. When pressed for specifics she confided, 'He often comes up to bed later than me, and in the morning I discover that he –' she whispered – 'has *forgotten to put the dishwasher on*.'

Adam had to suppress his smile, for her concern was real and frightening for her and needed more exploration. Alone the dishwasher failure is not worrying, but Adam checked there had not been other more significant lapses.

For someone concerned about dementia, for themselves or someone else, the first step is to take a breath and move beyond 'we didn't like to say it'. GPs and geriatricians take worries about dementia seriously. There are medical jobs to do. Occasionally it turns out that something else is going on, mimicking dementia but more treatable. For Margaret we'll check her thyroid hormones and look at her vitamin B12 and calcium levels. We'll make sure she's not depressed, as this can mess up anyone's ability to think. Often, even when someone does have dementia, there may be things making it worse – we need to treat Margaret's infection and make sure that none of her medications are slowing her brain. Drug side effects can be subtle, and it's not always the obvious medicines like strong painkillers that cause trouble; increasingly we're recognizing that tablets given for quite different problems can deplete the brain of the important chemicals it needs. We look out for tablets prescribed for overactive bladder and sleeping tablets and medicines given for anxiety. Depression makes dementia worse, but some antidepressants can do so too; there are fine balancing acts to be performed.

A diagnosis also opens the door to treatments. The tablets for Alzheimer's disease, boosting levels of acetylcholine, can slow the disease. For a few people they make a startling difference; for others the effect is marginal but still useful, and although we don't have firm evidence it seems likely that medications started early in the illness may be more effective than those started later. The same medicines sometimes make a substantial difference to the 'brain fog' of those who have dementia with Lewy bodies, and may also banish hallucinations and improve unsteadiness. Dementia drugs don't work for everyone, and they don't work for ever, but they are usually worth a try.

However, there's a reason perhaps better than any of these for finding the words to say to ourselves 'I am worried about my memory, and I think it may be more than just getting older', or to one another, 'I am worried about your memory, because it doesn't seem as sharp as it was', and then finding the courage to take these words to our GP. There is a pressing need to find the words to ask for help, and to be heard when we ask for that help.

Andrew described his parents' experience. 'Mum took Dad to the clinic, and I asked her after what they'd said, but she was a bit hazy, just that they were kind and all that, but Dad didn't like it. They were nice enough, they did some tests, and asked did he want to know any more, and he said no, and Mum thought he was tired, so they came home. And when I was next down she showed me the letter Dad got, which said all about his score on the tests and that he had problems with his memory, but it didn't actually say he had dementia, just that he didn't want to discuss the diagnosis, and didn't want to go to a memory club or whatever, so they discharged him. And that feels a bit tough on Mum, because she's the one doing all the work and all the worrying, and she's left wondering, well . . . does he have it or not?'

His story is not unusual: clinic staff are respectful of their patients' wishes, but as Andrew observed, 'Dad doesn't realize it would help my mother if she just knew.' Without a diagnosis doors may be closed to Andrew's mum; many support services, fearful of being over-whelmed, won't help the carers of those who haven't been given a formal dementia label. Yet Andrew's mum was affected by more than just missing out on practical advice about claiming carer's allowance, or accessing the 'sitting services' provided by voluntary groups.

The formulation of a dementia diagnosis is often nuanced, tentative; without a specific test everything rests on the story, and often we have not yet heard enough of each story to know what it will be about. We may have to wait six months, a year, and observe wors-ening behaviour or memory to see the story's true subject declare itself. In the meantime we may need to shelter behind woolly phrases: 'cognitive impairment', 'memory problems', 'short-term memory loss'. Sometimes these phrases genuinely mean that we have recognized that there may be a problem but that we cannot yet pin it down. Often, though, the diagnosis is obvious, the necessary assessments are complete, and the euphemisms really mean 'We know this person has dementia but we're not talking about it'.

I know Andrew's parents: they are a private, modest couple. I can see that without a diagnosis his mother is unable to explain to her friends why her husband's behaviour has become unsettling, rude even – or why their phone is unanswered or why she no longer attends the senior citizens' outings. And that is where medical teams go badly wrong, and it isn't fair. If professionals can't talk about it, can't work out a way to share this diagnosis sensitively and truthfully, then we give the impression that having dementia is not only difficult and unlucky, but also shameful. Shame is the very last emotion we should allow those with dementia and their families to suffer. Shame has no role in this condition.

Some years ago I sat with a group of trainee geriatricians at a conference. Two had recently returned from Tanzania, where they had been setting up a project in rural villages to evaluate rates of disability and dementia. 'How did you work out who had dementia?' I asked. They were full of energy, these young doctors. 'Well, that was a big challenge,' they told me. 'We couldn't use a standard screen like the AMT.' The Abbreviated Mental Test, devised in 1972 by Henry Hodkinson and familiar to generations of geriatricians, includes questions about date of birth, the years of the First (or Second) World War, the current monarch.

'In the end we came up with some formal questions, but when we started we worked out that the best thing was to just ask people is there anyone in this village who used to be someone you would go to for advice, but you wouldn't ask their advice any more?'

I've thought about those doctors and their Tanzanian colleagues often since, their dedication to discovery, their verve. Then I picture that old man or woman far away in a village, sitting at the door of a hut where the surrounding sand is swept smooth for the deterrence of snakes, and I wonder whether shame is allowed to colour the diagnosis of dementia in that society too, and I feel terribly sad. It seems such a waste, so unreasonable a way for a life to end, a life that has been filled with experience and learning, to have been once a wise person and now no longer wise. To compound that slow loss of wisdom, of personality, by allowing dementia to be something shameful – that is very wrong.

Dementia is a stigmatized condition, and we need to sort that out. Instead of shame we must harness the positive emotional fuels of change: compassion, a sense of angry injustice or pragmatic determination. These are the powerful emotions that inspire campaigns for better care, raise funds for research programmes or allow us to find one more sweet drop of patience at the end of a long day – emotions that may help us in our response to the diagnosis of dementia.

*

I think the best website for information about all kinds of dementia is that of the Alzheimer's Society:
https://www.alzheimers.org.uk/

10. Responding to Dementia

It's the Christmas holidays, and we've been having lunch with the Peters family. Cousins have arrived from the north, and Granny P has come for the day too. She has brought her dog, an elderly spaniel with a broad back and clouded eyes; he's lying patiently on a beaten-up sofa, having his ears chewed by the new puppy. There are twenty-two of us for lunch; chairs have been brought down from bedrooms, a piano stool's been dragged into the kitchen, and the three smallest children are wedged together on the windowsill. Everyone's excited – the house is warm and noisy, the older teenagers have found the cider, the little ones are high on 7 Up, and the red wine delivers an inky smack. Ham and leek pie, peas, leftover cranberry sauce. Blackberry and apple crumble is being demolished when Tom stands and announces, 'We're playing Empires,' and there's a flurry as slips of paper are handed out and the pen jar is passed down the table.

'Right,' shouts Tom above the grumbles about empty biros and yellow pencils.

'Each choose yourself a country and write it on your bit of paper. Don't show anyone; put it in the bowl. And make sure I can read it please, Alice.'

Then there's staring into space and crossings-out and demands for fresh pieces of paper, and finally all the countries are in the bowl, and Tom shouts again. 'Ready? I'm going to read them all out. Only once, so listen up. Max, are you concentrating?'

Twenty-two countries are read out, and the game begins. Max is allowed to start.

'Granny P, are you the president of Mexico?' he asks.

And Granny P says, no, she is not the president of Mexico, so it's her turn, and she asks one of the cousins whether he is the president of Azerbaijan, which he is not; it's the cousin's turn to guess now, and the game goes on.

'Mum, are you the president of Papua New Guinea?' one of the children asks her mother, and it turns out that she is, so there's shuffling of seats, and places are exchanged, and Alice joins her daughter to form the beginning of an empire. There are whoops when a guess hits its mark, and one small empire merges with another.

'Granny P, might you be the president of Belgium?' one of her sons-in-law enquires, and there's an almost undetectable pause before Granny P says no, she is not the president of Belgium, and it's her turn again. One by one the countries are assigned to their presidents, and empires grow and are absorbed as their leaders are unveiled, until there are only two big empires, together with Max and Granny P, who has turned out also not to be the president of Portugal, nor Ecuador, nor the Turks and Caicos Islands.

One of the cousins confers with his empire, and Max is asked, 'Max, are *you* the president of Mexico?' Max groans with disappointment at being found out, and there's cheering, and the game is over because Alice announces that Granny P is the winner.

One of the cousins asks, 'Granny, which country were you anyway?'

Granny P beams, saying, 'What a good game. I did enjoy that very much.' She stands to help clear the table, and the children shout 'Thank you for lunch' as they rush outside.

Later, I scoop the slips of paper from the bowl. One unfolds in my palm, as I hear the clinks of washing-up and children playing football in the last of the light, its neat old-fashioned script reading 'Belgium'.

Granny P has been to the memory clinic recently, Tom told me, and has been given a diagnosis of Alzheimer's dementia. 'She's taken it very well,' he said. 'She just says, "Oh well, life goes on," and it feels as if she's probably right, because nothing's really changed. She's still OK at home, and I know we'll have to think about her driving at some point, and she'll need some more help, but for now she doesn't seem too worried. It's more us worrying, than her.'

Geriatricians see lots of people with dementia. Many of our patients have had symptoms for a long time – they and their families haven't sought advice, perhaps because they feel their memory difficulties are normal, or because it seems unlikely that anything can be done, or because they don't want to cause upset to someone they love, or because they are embarrassed or afraid – of being taken from their home or of being the person who has 'lost her marbles'. For many it's only when they come into hospital with something else that the situation unravels and we question their family carefully and realize that, in fact, a diagnosis of dementia could have been made several years previously. At this stage our patients' awareness of their diagnosis may be fleeting; by the next day they have often forgotten our conversation, and may simply live in the moment once more, being reassured by a smile or a kindly voice, a conversation about tea or the weather. But much of the diagnostic work in dementia is done not by geriatricians but by psychogeriatricians, who run most dementia clinics. They tend to see people at an earlier stage of the disease and their outlook is perhaps rather different.

I spoke to my psychogeriatrician colleagues and asked them, 'What should someone actually do? If I was a patient, and I've just walked out of your clinic with that diagnosis, and I am wondering, well, what next? What do I do with that knowledge?'

John and Martin are kindly and experienced, and both told me much the same thing.

John explained, 'I think people have this awful perception of dementia because what you see on television is people at the end of the illness, people in care, and those who are clearly deranged and often distressed, and that makes a good *Panorama* image but it's not what life is like for many people.'

Martin agreed, adding, 'And also in the past the diagnosis was often made late, when people were indeed in rather a bad way, but we make the diagnosis so much earlier now; it's important that people know that actually lots of people do live with dementia, have pretty normal lives. It's not fair to put a gloss on it because it's still a diagnosis no one wants to hear, but we need to offer a balanced picture.'

Granny P's experience seemed to chime with what Martin and John have said. Tom told me, 'For the first few days after the clinic with Mum I felt as if we were ... I don't know, sliding down the Cresta Run, no brakes, really panicky. Then we realized that nothing had changed, and we just needed to calm down a bit and make some plans.'

What's going to happen next? John described how he explains the future to his patient and their family. 'I tend to "frame" the diagnosis, to keep it in perspective. I tell people that, in fact, only one in seven people diagnosed with dementia will die of it, so most people who have dementia don't actually reach that stage, you know, end-stage dementia.'

But Martin added, 'Yes, that can be a kind way to explain things, but I think it's fair to be clear that dementia is progressive; it does get worse. Obviously you have to judge carefully what information someone can handle, but the reason you don't die of dementia is because you'll probably die of something else first, especially if you're diagnosed when you're in your eighties or nineties.'

Both Martin and John emphasized the need for time to process the diagnosis. Martin said, 'I don't want people to leave my clinic feeling their life has ended. Actually, the shopping still needs doing, and chances are you'll do the shopping this week, after the diagnosis, just the same way you did the shopping last week. In the long run you'll need to make adjustments and have more help, but mostly things change slowly.'

They advocated taking time to plan. John was firm. 'I always say make a will, get your finances sorted out, have a talk with your family about Lasting Power of Attorney, both for the money side and the health and well-being bit.'

Martin agreed, saying, 'Yes, make clear plans, definitely talk with your family, don't hide it away from them,' but he added, 'and get on with it. Do things you enjoy! If you always promised you'd visit your sister in Australia, now's the time to do it. Don't put things off, do them now, enjoy them – build up a bank of happy memories.'

My patients who have dementia do not tend to ask questions about prognosis, 'How long have I got?' But their families do, understandably preparing themselves. It's hard to answer that question, because there's such variability. Even those diagnosed when they are young may be on a spiral of decline, though it's not unusual for someone diagnosed in their sixties and in otherwise good health to live for many years – fifteen or more. It doesn't always work out like that for older people, especially those who may be already frail when they are diagnosed with dementia. Startling data from the Netherlands, published in 2016, found that over-sixty-fives newly diagnosed with dementia were three to four times more likely to die over the next year compared with the general population; when the researchers looked at those who had been diagnosed with dementia during a hospital stay as well as those seen in clinic, one in three had died within a year (the data was collected around the time of legalization of euthanasia in the Netherlands, but before more than a handful of people had taken that route). In a study from a Chicago team, people newly diagnosed with Alzheimer's disease lived for just under four years on average – but that is an average, and the individual variation was wide.

Although some people with dementia seem to soldier on ('Mum's practically immortal,' one daughter told me), it is not unusual for things to go suddenly and irretrievably awry.

Renata had been diagnosed only recently. Just over a year ago she'd had a gall bladder infection and had become confused with delirium, and although the infection had cleared up with strong antibiotics her confusion had persisted. Around one in three people with delirium make a full recovery quite rapidly. Another third improve more slowly, but eventually get back to around the level they were at before the illness. And about one in three don't recover; for many an episode of delirium is the start of a slippery slope. Delirium is not a benign condition.

Renata had gone home after the gall bladder infection to her annex in the home of her son and daughter-in-law, where they had helped her with meals and cleaning, but her confusion hadn't got better and there had been a distressing episode when she became obsessed about money, stuffing bank statements into her blouse and clutching her handbag in bed at night. A year on, the memory team had diagnosed Alzheimer's disease, and had tried donepezil, but that seemed to make things worse, and she came back into hospital with another infection, this time a patch of pneumonia at the bottom of her left lung. Again, she had delirium and her behaviour fluctuated; there were hours of sleepy vagueness during which she sat head in hands, but she also had spells of restlessness. Her sodium level was low, a feature common in pneumonia, but it had been running a little below normal for a year for no obvious reason; we don't understand exactly why that happens, but it's often a hint that something's amiss with the brain. For Renata, once again, all the signs of infection melted away quickly on antibiotics – she barely had a fever, even at the start, and the markers of inflammation in her blood resolved quickly. She had copious blood tests to look for rarer causes of confusion, and a study of her brainwaves (an EEG) and scans of her brain and the rest of her body (occasionally a tumour hidden elsewhere can inexplicably cause a rapidly progressive confusion, a condition called a paraneoplastic phenomenon) but there was nothing to find. Renata went home once more, and came back six weeks later, this time flamboyantly confused, increasingly thin and unsteady. She was treated again for pneumonia, although her chest X-ray had improved. By now she had had several falls and more unremarkable brain scans; she went to a community hospital for rehabilitation but made no progress, and she became more withdrawn and did not respond to antidepressants. Her family tried having her at home again, juggling work, children and grandchildren, but Renata fell beside her bed one night and was back in hospital once more, on another course of antibiotics, when she died. The situation was miserable for Renata and her sons, and sad for those looking after her, who watched the progress of the dismal roller-coaster without having any control – there was no big lever to stop the ride.

We have a lot to learn about the interplay of delirium and dementia. We know that people who've had an episode of delirium in later life are more likely to develop dementia, and we know that delirium worsens dementia, but we don't know why. Is it that people whose brains are already vulnerable, because of a dementia that hasn't yet declared itself, are more likely to become confused? Or does the delirium itself cause the damage? And in which case how? Is it the chemical compounds, cytokines, released by immune system cells as they fight off infection, that inadvertently damage the brain? Does delirium due to things other than infection – chemical upsets or drugs – have the same deleterious effect? Is it some sort of stress response, raised cortisol levels, that messes up the brain's ability to produce its essential neurotransmitters? Even without episodes of delirium, dementia progresses faster in some than in others – why? And for someone like Renata, eighty-three when she first became unwell, strong-willed, warm-hearted creator of Portuguese family feasts – how much should we put her through in our search for something rare but possibly treatable? How can her family make sense of this senseless situation, respond to the tipping of the scales, when at first there were good days and hope, but later nothing good, no conversation, no 'Please can I have your recipe for *pastéis*?', nor 'Do you think, Grandma, that this will look nice on the baby?' And in this situation, which is not rare, some of the most difficult conversations need to take place, in which families may need to come to terms with loss faster than they feel able, and medical teams must be honest because the most likely explanation by far of Renata's decline is simply, sadly, dementia.

Sometimes a person has been able to throw his or her thoughts into the future and has been given a chance to articulate the hopes and fears therein through a conversation or a written plan, which I talk about in Chapter 13, and this is a great help to those who love them. Without such knowledge a family and a medical team need to share an uncertain dark journey and feel their way by degrees in an attempt to care for someone exactly as they would wish to be cared for. To do this, to feel we have cared for someone as well as we can, and in the way that they themselves would wish, is one of the most difficult challenges we face together.

Anna told me about her father, describing what had been happening at home in Sheffield. Her dad's memory was terrible – he needed help with the bills and with planning his vegetable planting and remembering appointments.

'Mum's doing everything now.' Anna was matter-of-fact. 'I think Dad's probably got dementia, but not, you know, *Alzheimer's.*'

I realized that she meant that he does indeed have dementia, and I know it probably *is* due to Alzheimer's disease, but he isn't troublesome; he doesn't accost strangers or have wild staring eyes or suddenly start to cry for no reason. He doesn't look like someone on the TV with Alzheimer's, who is anxious, apathetic, wanders or is physically challenging – Anna's dad doesn't have, yet, what are called 'behavioural and psychological symptoms of dementia', or BPSD, which are the next difficult thing to talk about and are a nest of snakes.

There are lots of moments in this book when I want to stop writing because I'm worried about how you are feeling. If we were together in a room, I'd be watching you all the time, listening to your responses; I'd be trying to read your expression, gauging whether this is the right information for you, or the right information but the wrong time. I'd try to choose good words for you, and maybe put a hand on yours, or not, or just sit for a moment together. I am aware that you may be reading this because dementia has stuck its ugly mean face into your life in some way, and I do not want you to feel alone. Perhaps we can think together about the hard problems with which this illness confronts us, and what might be done about them.

There are many features of BPSD; no one with dementia will get them all, but almost everyone will get some. More than memory loss, they are the symptoms that cause unhappiness and squeeze the hearts of those who mind about someone who has dementia. They can be made better or worse by how we respond to them; some can be helped by simple changes, minor adaptations of our own behaviour or the environment or by imaginative activities; others require serious decisions about risky medication. Some are made worse by our own reaction: repetitive behaviour or aggression, for example, may escalate when challenged head on. Some symptoms are difficult to overcome and need a different approach. And no one should ever be left to cope with the worst behavioural and psychological symptoms of dementia on their own.

The hospital inspectors, the Care Quality Commission (CQC) were visiting, and spent two days on our ward, flicking through notes, quizzing staff on hand hygiene, talking with visiting families and checking the underside of commode seats. Throughout their visit Marie, who was waiting to move into a care home, sat in D Bay, bellowing, 'Help! Help!', and one of us would go to her and say, 'Are you OK, Marie?' and she'd look up all smiling and say, 'Yes, I'm fine,' and we'd turn to another task and she'd start again. Calling out is a well-recognized behaviour, and once we have excluded some unmet need (perhaps something as simple as needing a pee), the evidence-based advice is to ignore the behaviour and instead to reward calm, quiet moments by stopping for a chat when someone is peaceful. Our prompt, reliable response to her calls, to reassure Marie (and the CQC team), may have been making her behaviour worse, but it's hard to get it right, to work out why Marie wants our attention and adapt our behaviour positively to encourage hers to change too, for in other instances someone may need to be listened to and to have their worries explored and validated.

For many things on the BPSD list there's an approach that may help, and finding it is the challenge. For those worrying about someone with bad dementia there are some things worth knowing.

It's worth knowing that agitation and restlessness may arise from a physical cause of distress. Worth knowing, for example, that older men get prostate trouble and may find it painfully impossible to pee, and occasionally being unable to pee happens to women too.

Worth knowing that constipation is a miserably under-recognized cause of uneasy behaviour in those with dementia, and that diarrhoea in the most frail or muddled people is paradoxically very often caused by constipation, a condition called overflow. Worth knowing that pain in those with dementia may be inexpressible, except by a change in behaviour; we must look out for sore joints or an aching tooth. Dementia specialists recognize that surprisingly often distressed behaviour can be relieved simply by regular paracetamol.

After that, it's a matter of thinking is it a new environment, or over-stimulation, noise or lights, or maybe sadness or boredom? One February day, the ward's activity coordinator, Mandy, was tasked with looking after Alf. Fearless and determined, he kept darting unsteadily towards the door, tapping his forefinger threateningly on the chest of anyone who stood in his way. I love Mandy; she read the information that had come from his care home and disappeared for a while, before setting Alf up with a basin of potatoes and a peeler. 'Army Catering Corps,' Mandy told me, and Alf sat all afternoon peeling potatoes, turning them slowly in his sinewy hands until they were perfect.

Many people who live with someone who has dementia, and the best care home staff, respond to difficult behaviours almost instinctively. The restless are included in tasks: gardening, making beds or folding clean towels, and they sleep better too for having had a busy day. The apathetic may be lifted by music or an art activity; the depressed by a trip to a park, the seaside. Restlessness and calling out are among the symptoms that respond best to imaginative activities like Mandy's. But there are other symptoms, pervasive, draining behaviours, that exhaust carers. Sometimes symptoms respond to clever adjustments to care and environment or to medication; sometimes they do not. Delusions, hallucinations, disturbed sleep, screaming, depression – this is a grim list and it goes on. Repetitive activities, disinhibition, sexual behaviours, anxiety, agitation. These are symptoms that often tip the balance, shatter the scales completely; they cause households to break down and precipitate a move into care. They fuel guilt and despair, and cause us to have thoughts that we feel unable to share. We may feel desperately alone, and yet none of us are alone, because someone else has also had these thoughts, is having them now, and we need to be in this together in our response to dementia.

A tall woman stood at the nurses' station. She was wearing a dusty-pink linen jumper and a brown flowing skirt with pink flowers, a wide belt sitting loosely on her slim hips. Several gold necklaces rested on her chest, and her fine silver hair curled neatly round her ears and at the nape of her neck. She closed her eyes and her hand reached for the shelf of the station and I moved towards her, thinking she was about to fall, but she shook her head and breathed in deeply through her nose and looked at me.

'May I talk to you about my husband?'

I hadn't seen Clem yet, but I knew he was out for the count, having been given a hefty sedative downstairs in ED. The admission note said *worsening confusion – social crisis* and I had just been looking at the electronic records kept by the dementia team.

Nancy and I sat on a beige leatherette sofa while she told me about Clem. His war years and his time in a POW camp about which he rarely spoke. His military service after the war in countries that were struggling towards democracy. Clem's medals, his UN work. His affection for their children, his wry humour and his love for her – Nancy's hand moved to hold a lumpy pale pink stone, quartz maybe, that was set in gold on one of her necklaces. Clem had had dementia for four years. To begin with he was filled with self-loathing, berating himself for memory lapses. He had become depressed and spoke of suicide, and over the last two years he had developed 'visions – hallucinations, dreams, memories? I don't know', terrifying images that caused him to start and shout. They'd tried assorted dementia drugs, but nothing worked. Clem would pace the house at night, pulling things from cupboards and fiddling with the front-door lock.

Nancy continued her story, words spilling. Her hands were together now, rubbing over and over each other on her lap. Clem had accused her of having an affair, many affairs, of keeping men hidden in the house. He had spent a while in the psychiatric hospital; he'd had his ninetieth birthday while he was there, and his medicines had been changed again. He'd come home last week and she'd thought it was going to be better, but this morning he had picked up a knife from the side in the kitchen, a little knife with a brown handle, and had held it to her throat.

Nancy twisted towards me and she grabbed my wrist and brought her face close to mine and whispered, 'I *long* for him to die,' before letting go, throwing her hands over her face. She made no sound, but I could see tears squeezing out between the rings on her fingers, and all I could do was hold her, hold this graceful, composed woman and feel her thin shoulder blades, and say, 'It's fine. It's fine. It's OK to feel like that,' over and over again.

Many people who have dementia are contented and are cherished. They entertain and can be entertained. Their lives are good and good-humoured and are valued by themselves and those around them. But this is not true for everyone, and even with the best care there are some for whom living with dementia entails unrelenting, unmendable suffering. I do not think it is wrong in such circumstances to love someone and to wish for their death at the same time.

How *do* people with dementia die? As John my psychogeriatrician colleague pointed out, most people with dementia die of something else. For those who die of dementia itself the illness produces a gradual withdrawal from the world, a reduction of interest in people and pastimes, and eventually the life of someone who has dementia is focused on very basic needs – eating, drinking. And with time even these activities lose their interest. A mouthful of food is swallowed, but the next mouthful is not taken from the spoon, or is held, unacknowledged, on the tongue, and a daughter may say, 'Come on, Mum, swallow that down,' and nothing happens. This can be very hard for families, who see that without food or drink there cannot be life, and they might wonder should Mum have a tube to feed her, but this has been shown to be of no benefit to those at the end of the dementia journey – tube feeding does not prolong life in this illness. It feels perhaps as if the person who has dementia is receding from us, their body forgets that life requires us to eat, and at the very end their lungs forget to breathe and their heart forgets to beat.

For most people who have dementia, however, a different illness comes along that threatens their life, and some perhaps feel that this represents an opportunity for themselves rather than a threat. Clem had been treated earlier that year for a bout of sepsis, transferring from the psychiatric hospital to the general hospital one night, with antibiotics administered through a drip, on the assumption that such treatment was right and essential.

There are legitimate conversations to be had about treatments that should not be withheld just because someone has dementia, and, conversely, treatments that might be entirely unwanted because of that illness, and the balance will be different for each person. So as well as holding Nancy, later she and I sit together and make a plan for Clem's future care that reflects the situation that he is in and the wishes of the man to whom she has been married for sixty-seven years.

What should our response be to dementia? We don't understand it – we need far more research into both delirium and dementia. We are ashamed of it – we need to share information, to learn and fight stigma, banish shame. We fear it – we need advice and help from professionals, who must be well trained, have time and understand what might be done to alleviate distress. Dementia makes us feel guilty – we need to be held, to know that we are not alone. Dementia tries to take away love – we need to pour love back into those whose capacity for love seems exhausted.

I was on my way home from work one Monday when I dropped in to one of the wards to visit Noel; he was a friend of my mother's, a retired academic, and Mum had heard he was in hospital. Noel was a historian, and in youth had an impressive amateur sporting career. The ward sister told me he was doing well and was due to go home tomorrow. Noel's son Mark was visiting and greeted me; I perched on the bed while Mark explained, 'We were just talking about the rugby yesterday, weren't we, Dad?'

Noel nodded and grinned – he looked like Wallace with cheese – and said, 'It was a bus, tree.'

To which Mark replied, 'They played very well, didn't you think?'

Noel smiled, saying, 'Any Rome, the main thing, the towel . . .' before tailing off and smiling again, raising his eyebrows to Mark, who lifted his hands into a rugby-ball-throwing position, and said, 'Brilliant how they fizzed the ball down that line.' And he flicked his wrists and Noel raised his hands too, which were huge beautiful hands ready to catch that ball, and his eyes sparkled.

As Mark and I walked to the car park I asked about his conversation with his father.

Mark explained, 'I used to get so frustrated; I'd mention the cricket, or the rugby, but it was so obvious that he couldn't remember what had happened, even just the day after, and for a while I didn't talk about it at all because it was too depressing. Then I met someone, a nurse, when I took him to clinic, and I watched him just chatting nonsense with her, and he looked so happy, and none of it made any sense but she didn't seem to mind. And I realized that often when I was talking with Dad I was sort of *testing* his memory, and that wasn't helping him. Or me. I've worked out how to do it now; it doesn't always work and I'm not sure whether he's remembering . . . I don't know, some match in 1980 or whether he knows what we're talking about at all, but it doesn't matter.'

I've had many conversations with those who have dementia and I am aware that these are often not conversations about any real past, because memories are blurred, or about the future. That's very hard for those who are with them day in, day out, who cannot live in the present alone. It's hard too for the daughter I met on a train going to visit her mother. 'A two-hour train journey for a half-hour visit she won't remember the minute I've left.'

Mark and I stood at the entrance of the multistorey, and he went on. 'Mum's amazing. I don't know how she does it; she just manages to be in the moment with him.'

I think I understand what Mark means. His mother Sally has to recall the past with accuracy, noting that the car's last MOT was in November, and she must think about the future and plan for Noel's audiology appointment next week, and send a birthday card to a grandchild, while working out how to be contented with Noel just where he is right now.

Mark looked past me, back up to the second floor of the red-brick hospital, where his father would be having a sandwich and a mug of soup, and he continued, a little uncertainly. 'It's . . . well, it's a bit like mindfulness. You have to forget the past and the future, and just sit in the present. In the present he's happy. And actually so am I. We are both happy.'

*

Here is the Dutch study about prognosis:
https://bmjopen.bmj.com/content/5/10/e008897

And here is the Chicago one:
https://www.ncbi.nlm.nih.gov/pubmed/24598707/

There's a great Canadian educational resource about BPSD. It's designed for medics and has a lot of technical detail, but may also be useful to those caring for people with BPSD:
https://www.psychdb.com/geri/dementia/1-bpsd

11. Driving

I was on the phone to my friend Laura. We were at university together, but she's a teacher and lives miles away, and we rarely see one another. After a long download of the adventures of our children, I asked after her mum. Laura paused, and sighed.

'I'm worried sick about her.'

'What's up?'

'I don't want to make you do work outside work . . .'

'It's fine, what's the worry?'

'It's her driving.'

Laura's mum Connie had lived on her own since her husband Paddy died. She was lively and determined; Connie had trained as a vet many years ago, when women didn't train to be vets, and since retiring she'd thrown herself into other passions – the creation of exuberant oil paintings and open-water swimming competitions, until her farmer's lung kicked in. She was a lot of fun.

'Tell me everything.'

'It's just . . . oh, awful.' I could hear Laura filling the kettle, could picture her moving around her kitchen, phone propped between shoulder and ear, getting supper ready.

'Her eyes are fine, and the heart people said it was OK for her to drive, but it's not really a medical problem, I think. It's more her judgement. You know what her driving's like.'

For a moment I was back in Connie's car the first time I met her, over thirty years ago. She had collected Laura and me from the station, hungover after finishing our second-year exams. We sped along the top road towards their small town between walls of once golden stone, now darkened by the soot of the industrial revolution; the windows were down and clouds scudded in the bright sky above the moor. The road swept into a valley, and Connie's fair hair blew around her head as she shouted, 'Whizzer bridge coming up, hold on to your tummies,' and I saw Laura's hand reach up to grab her seat belt, and the car accelerated, flying over the bridge, and I could taste yesterday's vodka at the back of my throat.

Laura was still talking, cutlery chinking as she laid the table. 'She doesn't judge spaces right, the car is covered in bashes and scratches. She says, "Oh, someone drove into it when I was in Morrisons," which is just a fib; I know it was her reversing into something. And she keeps a little pot of paint in the glovebox to cover up the new marks so she thinks I don't see them.'

I smiled. 'And?'

'And she's got very naughty about parking; she basically just puts it where she wants. She's got a blue badge because she's so breathless, but, honestly, the kids came back from town the other day and they'd taken a picture of her car on the pavement outside the post office – I mean, all four wheels were on the pavement. It's just embarrassing.'

I snorted.

'I know it should be funny, Luce, but it's not, because the worst thing is the speed; she's done the speed-awareness course twice, but she hasn't slowed down, and I know her reflexes just aren't as quick. I'm so worried she's going to hit someone, and other people are too – someone rang me from her church the other day saying they were worried about the Sunday-school kids because she roars up late, and they asked me to stop her from driving, and I tried but she just says she'll go to a different church.'

Oh, Connie. Now that is bad behaviour.

'Do you think she might be getting dementia?' I asked.

'I'm not sure. She might be. She's clever, and she's still very active, but . . . you know what she's like; she was never very good about appointments and that kind of thing, but it's definitely worse. Actually, thinking about it, she's getting to be a bit like a teenager. She's never quite where I think she's going to be, and she doesn't answer her phone or pass on messages. And she's got sloppy about washing-up, and her house is a bit of a dive.'

After our conversation I thought about what Laura had said. There was plenty of love in there, but also worry, and now exasperation. Connie's domestic arrangements may have raised an eyebrow, but they were her business, and one of the good things about getting older is a freedom from the social norms by which younger generations feel bound. Jenny Joseph's poem 'Warning', announcing her intention to wear purple and run her stick along public railings, became popular for good reason, and Connie's erratic diary-keeping was forgiven by her friends, who laughed when she turned up for lunch unexpectedly. It was her close family, her children, who were going to be most bothered by Connie's behaviour, and as my colleague Peter says, 'It can be a bit like helicopter parenting, except directed up a generation. People need to learn to leave their parents to get on with it.'

But driving is different. Laura's concern was for the safety of others as well as her mum. Laura felt that she needed to do something, that she must assume responsibility, at least in part, for her mum's dangerous driving, and her feeling was exacerbated by other people phoning her to complain.

Is it fair to regard driving as a potential problem? Why is it that news headlines mention the age of a driver who has been in an accident only if they are very young – a teenager – or much older? *Elderly couple involved in crash. Eighty-year-old driver in motorway nightmare.* No headline announces *Fifty-three-year-old in dual carriage smash* or *Middle-aged man causes road chaos.* Each report implies that an older driver has had an accident, not in the way other people have accidents, because of ice or a burst tyre, but because they are old. Every report of the Duke of Edinburgh's car crash in 2019 commented on his age (then ninety-seven), and even the most deferential royal watchers suggested it was time for Prince Philip to hand in his keys. Yet older drivers are potentially safer than young ones, as they are less likely to take risks such as driving too fast or while distracted, and statistics bear this out; they are less commonly involved in speed-related accidents or caught texting at the wheel. But above eighty, while the actual number of older drivers involved in accidents doesn't seem much different from the young, their *rate* of involvement is higher, as there are fewer of them. And the older driver tends to make shorter journeys, so data from the US suggests that for drivers over eighty the number of accidents *per mile travelled* is higher. They are more likely to be involved in incidents where judging distance and speed is important, such as when turning on to a busy road. And if they are involved in an accident, people over seventy-five are much more likely than a younger driver to die as a result.

Older people don't generally need lectures about their safety behind the wheel. They come to their own conclusions, noting their hesitation at a junction, the uncomfortable squint into the sun, the near miss at a roundabout; most older drivers are good, safe drivers and instinctively know when to stop. But not all.

For families and friends, knowing when to step in when someone's driving seems unsafe is a big problem, and knowing how is even bigger. Driving, so inter-twined with independence, is an emotive issue.

It's easier when the rules are clear. The Driver and Vehicle Licensing Agency, DVLA (or Driver and Vehicle Agency (DVA) in Northern Ireland), has stark rules about many medical conditions. No driving for four weeks after heart-valve surgery, or for one month after a mini-stroke. Everything is laid out in detail: *For an episode of loss of consciousness while sitting, with an identifiable trigger, driving may resume after four weeks only if the cause has been identified and treated.* For many conditions the guidance is rightly uncompromising. There are strict, specific measurements governing the acceptable levels of vision, and the rules are unsurprisingly fiercer for the drivers of buses and lorries.

However, the guidance covering changes in cognition, with its effects on judgement or insight, is necessarily vaguer, and there is no guidance at all about simply getting older, which leaves people like Laura in a difficult situation.

When someone has been diagnosed with dementia the rules are straightforward, although their implementation may not be. I talked with Martin; as a psychogeriatrician he's spent years guiding his patients and their families through the intricacies of driving regulation.

Martin explained, 'The rules with dementia are clear. The DVLA must be notified, and technically it's the driver's own responsibility to do that. But that can be

quite hard for people who have dementia, just that business of getting organized and writing a letter, so I often
say, "Would you like me to let the DVLA know for
you?" and a lot of people are happy with that.'

Martin went on. 'Many folk just decide to stop driving then; most people are pretty good about it. They're
sad, but they take it on the chin. And if it's obvious they
shouldn't be driving, I will say that, but for others I
make it clear that they may still be able to drive if they
want to, but they'll probably be asked to take a test. There
are those, maybe with earlier stages of dementia, who
are still pretty good drivers, and the DVLA understand
that, so I can write a report saying, "This chap has
trouble with memory, but his coordination and reflexes
look good, and his judgement at the moment is OK."
You don't need a brilliant memory to be a good driver.'

I think of my friend Ally's dad driving confidently
around the Midlands, his judgement so far unimpaired
even though his specific, rare semantic dementia means
that he can no longer find the words for 'diesel', 'traffic
light' and 'slip road'.

Martin continued. 'And the DVLA will most probably arrange a test, and if he does OK, he is still allowed
to drive, and they check each year that he remains safe.'

I asked Martin about those who refuse to accept his
advice, who decline his offer to contact the DVLA and
refuse to do so themselves. I've talked with my own
patients about this, as I used to do a clinic for those who
had fallen, and many of my patients had episodes of loss

of consciousness, which for some meant not being allowed to drive for considerable lengths of time while we tracked down a cause. Most people were gracious about this, but occasionally I would notice a sideways look in my patient's eyes, perhaps towards the door, beyond which was the corridor, the entrance lobby, the car park, the car, and a wife sitting beside him, whose hands turned over one another in her lap.

Martin sighed. 'Ah, now that's where it gets thorny. People who don't have insight. It's not just whether someone is able to realize that he may not be a safe driver now; some people aren't able to accept that they may ever develop a problem. They don't see that an illness like dementia may make them unsafe. The chaps who say, "I've been driving for fifty years; no one is telling me what to do." They're not trying to be difficult. Sometimes they're stubborn fellows, but often it's the dementia itself that has robbed them of insight. That is more awkward.'

Martin and I talked about confidentiality, one of the pillars of medical practice in the UK and many other countries. The General Medical Council (GMC) explains: *Trust is an essential part of the doctor–patient relationship and confidentiality is central to this. Patients may avoid seeking medical help, or may under-report symptoms, if they think that their personal information will be disclosed by doctors without consent.*

The GMC also understands that confidentiality is not an absolute principle. *Doctors owe a duty of confidentiality to their patients, but they also have a wider duty to protect and promote the health of patients and the public.*

Yet confidentiality is closely guarded, and even in the matter of driving with dementia the GMC guidance is clear: doctors must think twice before abandoning this principle. We must consider whether a driver's refusal to stop driving, or even to inform the DVLA, *'leaves others exposed to a risk of death or serious harm'*.

Martin said, 'I don't find this too difficult. One of my patients years ago was a man with terrible depression – his son had been killed in an accident because of someone who shouldn't have been driving. It's people who don't have insight into their limitations who are most likely to be dangerous. I explain to them this isn't going to be my decision; what I am doing is letting the DVLA know and seeking their expert advice. I explain they will get a fair assessment, but if they won't tell the DVLA about their diagnosis, then I must do that. Again, I emphasize it's not my decision; it's the DVLA's decision.'

Martin's view is reiterated in the GMC's advice to doctors. *The Driver and Vehicle Licensing Agency (DVLA) in England, Scotland and Wales and the Driver and Vehicle Agency (DVA) in Northern Ireland are legally responsible for deciding if a person is medically unfit to drive. This means they need to know if a person holding a driving licence has a condition or is undergoing treatment that may now, or in the future, affect their safety as a driver.*

The DVLA's guidance states that in those who have dementia *lack of insight and judgement almost certainly mean no fitness to drive.* The guidance uses the same phrase about lack of insight to raise concerns about those who do not have dementia but instead have mild cognitive impairment (MCI), which is very common. And here the water is muddier as there is no statutory requirement to inform the DVLA of the diagnosis, even though some people with MCI are not safe to drive. And there is no guidance at all for those who are simply slowing up.

'How do I know,' asked my worried aunt, 'whether I'm a good driver or a bad driver with no insight?' and I reassured her that the fact that she was concerned about this at all probably meant that she was a good driver, and I told her about Bridget.

Bridget is my friend Juliet's mother, and has made careful plans about driving. Every so often Juliet hops into the passenger seat when Bridget is going shopping. Juliet watches but does not intervene, explaining, 'It doesn't help if I just back-seat drive, because it puts Mum on edge, and anyway I'm not with her the rest of the time. If she needs a co-pilot, someone pointing out hazards or signs or whatever, she shouldn't be driving.'

Bridget only uses familiar roads to the hairdresser and to Tesco and the butchers, and she and Juliet have changed her route, which had included a nasty right turn on to a busy road with limited visibility; cars come up fast round a corner from the left, and no one really likes that junction. They tested another way to town – it's a little longer but cuts out the dodgy turning. And Bridget gets her eyes tested and doesn't drive at night or in the rain, and they've talked about what she will do when she can't drive any more, so that it's not a sudden shock.

Bridget herself tells me, 'I don't even really like driving, but it'll be such a nuisance when I can't. So I make myself drive, and I know that if Juliet doesn't feel safe to get in my car, it's time for me to call it a day.'

Many people like Bridget worry about whether they are still driving safely, and they put the safety of others above their own independence. They may have a minor accident or hear of a friend's misfortune at the wheel and feel shaken; they lose faith in the strength of an arthritic hand on the steering wheel or the speed of a foot on a brake. It can be helpful then to have an objective test to restore confidence.

Various organizations provide driving assessments and advice. Driving Mobility is the umbrella group for many of them. The Driving Mobility team is sensitive to the importance of driving, and their website has sensible advice both about continuing to drive and retirement from driving. The older drivers I have met who have put themselves through their tests have told me they are thorough and considerately delivered, useful and fair.

Other drivers may need a nudge to consider their safety. Matt told me how he'd tackled the issue with his father, whose memory and judgement were subtly waning. 'I just kept telling him how proud I'd always been of his good driving – how when I was young I felt happy in his car. He was good at overtaking! And I said I didn't want to have that memory taken away by some stupid thing happening now, and eventually one day he said, "There's too many nutters on the road. I'm stopping while the going's good." '

But Laura was in a trickier position. Her mother Connie had no formal diagnosis of dementia, or even of mild cognitive impairment, and had no insight into her dangerous driving. She'd always driven as if she owned the road and had no intention of stopping now. Parking restrictions and speed limits had long represented only tentative suggestions to Connie, and if she wanted a loaf of bread, a loaf of bread she would have, regardless of whether she brought the town to a standstill. Connie was not a bad person; she'd have been devastated if she had harmed someone, but she just didn't believe that could happen.

A few months later, Laura and I talked again about Connie. Other warning signs had developed.

'I was behind her at a junction; she hesitated for ages even though there wasn't anything coming,' said Laura. 'I've a feeling she may have been fiddling with the radio. Then she shot across the road, by which time there was another car, and he had to brake pretty hard, and I don't think she even noticed.'

Laura had spoken with Connie's GP, who had said he'd have a word with her, but nothing seemed to happen and there were other bumps and scrapes, and Laura tried again, roping her brother into the conversation.

Connie said, 'I'll drive more carefully' and 'I won't listen to the radio while I'm driving' and 'I'll slow down before the thirty sign instead of at it', but nothing changed and Laura had fielded more distress calls from neighbours, and Connie's wing mirrors were held on with gaffer tape. In the end things came to a head.

'One of Mum's friends contacted the DVLA,' said Laura, 'and he asked me to do it too. He'd seen her have a near miss on the main road, and he said she'd never stop driving unless someone makes her, and he told me you could do a confidential report to the DVLA. I had to fill in a form online and put all the details in it. I'm waiting to hear what'll happen next.'

Driving is a privilege, not a right. It's also a lifeline for many, and without a car older people can become isolated and may miss out on activities that bring joy: church, clubs, visiting friends, days out. Public transport, especially in rural areas, may be a poor substitute; near Connie there's no bus back from the big town after five thirty. It takes over an hour to reach the nearest railway station. There's no bus to the cinema or the supermarket; there's an erratic service, with an unreliable change at the depot, to get to the hospital. There are no buses at all on Sundays. Without her car Connie would be dependent on taxis; she could use the money saved by not running a car, but her car was small and economical, and a taxi from her town to the big town would cost £31 each way, so would quickly drain her driving fund. Or she could use the community transport, but that needed planning in advance, and didn't go where Connie wanted to go to. Or she would be dependent on friends. Or on Laura.

I caught up with Laura again.

'Mum had the test,' she said. 'She was cross because they wouldn't let her do it in her own car, and I had to take her, and I felt so guilty because I was complicit in making her have a test. But it was so fair! They were very kind, and they did lots of checks, first her eyesight and then some thinking stuff, patterns, sorting things.'

There's no mental test that is completely reliable at predicting who will be safe or unsafe behind a wheel, and many will need an assessment on the road as well.

Laura continued. 'Then they took her out in a car, dual control – I'm not surprised – and she drove a bit in the test centre, then they went out with her on to the road, and they gave her a proper assessment. And they were very tactful but completely firm, saying she obviously had been good at it in the past, but her reflexes were letting her down, and they said they would issue a full report but they could tell she shouldn't be driving. It's such a relief. They didn't ask me anything. It was taken completely out of my hands.'

Families and our patients often have a perception that it is their doctor who will tell them when they should not drive, and that isn't the case. We can tell people what the DVLA rules are and can let them know when they have a condition that bars them from driving or that must be notified. We can offer advice to stop driving based on what we have seen or been told, and many people will accept that advice, but in the end the principle of confidentiality may mean that when there isn't a medical problem that fits the DVLA guidance – when the issue is with insight or judgement – the doctor is not the person who can intervene. Families and friends are not bound by confidentiality rules and can tell the DVLA their worries, and the DVLA is able to arrange an objective assessment. I think that seems fair.

*

Driving Mobility is a charity supported by the Department for Transport, which offers assessments for experienced older drivers who may have concerns about their standard of driving:

https://www.drivingmobility.org.uk/

There's very good advice on driving with dementia on the Alzheimer's Society website:

https://www.alzheimers.org.uk/get-support/staying-independent/driving-and-dementia

12. Decisions

'In the event of my being in a state in which I do not have capacity to make decisions about my care, and from which the chance of recovery is minimal, I do not wish to have life-sustaining treatment; this would include artificial nutrition and hydration, for example via a feeding tube. Such states would include vegetative or minimally conscious states, or other conditions like severe dementia, in which I am unable to communicate meaningfully with those I love. I would like to receive care directed at the alleviation of suffering and would expect to be offered food and drink by mouth, even if this might increase the risk of infections such as pneumonia. I understand that this advance decision to refuse treatment may have – is indeed likely to have – the effect of shortening my life.'

I wrote this on a piece of lined paper pulled from a notebook on 30 December 2014, a few months after my forty-ninth birthday. I've signed and dated it, and it's witnessed by my husband's signature; it is signed again, dated and witnessed, in 2016 and 2018. It lived for several years in my desk before being replaced by a more detailed successor. My husband and a friend know where to find it, my valid, legally binding advance decision to refuse treatment.

Why write such a thing? At the time my hospital's ethics committee had once again been approached by a team seeking help in making a decision about whether to place a permanent PEG feeding tube. This time it was the diabetes team who had come to us, but their patient didn't have diabetes. Rather, Esther was a woman in her forties with terrible problems relating to abuse, and subsequent drug and alcohol addiction. She had been in and out of hospital over many years. Esther had collected brain haemorrhages during drinking sprees, was paralysed down one side, and could speak only a few words. She lived in a care home that specialized in looking after adults with similar injuries. She had attempted suicide several times – the latest attempt, by hanging, had resulted in further damage to her brain and she now was unable to speak at all or to swallow. She'd been treated for severe pneumonia twice and pushed away nurses as they cared for her. She pulled out feeding tubes that had been placed through her nose into her stomach, even when these were tethered in place by a loop passed in through one nostril and out through the other. Attempts to communicate by means other than speech had failed; Esther's gestures were consistent only in the degree of anger they seemed to convey. Esther's steadfast, sweet-tempered girlfriend Rachel told the team of her love for the music of Nina Simone, and that she'd 'wanted to be dead every day for years'. And yet the arguments swayed back and forth. She was only forty-three. Who might say what her future could hold?

Her quality of life might be improved – a different care home, more music, an additional antidepressant.

Esther's case was one of many. The ethics committee had recently discussed ninety-seven-year-old Frank, a retired art dealer, who was unable to communicate following a major stroke. He had survived the first two weeks but had made little recovery, and his daughters were at Shakespearean loggerheads about whether he should continue to be fed by tube. One daughter described his zest for life, how when she visited the ward and put headphones on her father to pour Sibelius into his ears he would smile. The other daughter scorned her sister's assessment. 'That's not a smile; it's a grimace.'

The first daughter hissed back, 'It was a smile until *you* got here.'

The committee takes referrals from other hospitals. We had listened to the story of Helga, who had lived for two years in a nursing home, following a cardiac arrest with successful resuscitation but a poor recovery. She had not spoken nor eaten – sustained by a PEG feeding tube, she had at first walked a little around the home, but after a further heart attack she'd become weaker. The staff used a hoist to lift her between her bed and a chair. Her family had been ambivalent about the tube in the first place, unsure whether it was what she would have wanted, and now it had cracked and was leaking. Its proposed replacement would require Helga to come into hospital for a day and to be sedated for an endoscopy. Her sons baulked – they explained that in retrospect they felt guilty that they had not spoken out more force-fully against the placement of the tube when it was first being considered. Two years on, they felt this was not a life – doubly incontinent, silent and immobile – that their mother would have wanted. But Helga's carers and the GP who visited the home were sure that she was contented. Helga's house had been sold to pay for her care; there was a hint, never explicitly stated, that her family may have become fed up with authorizing hefty bank transfers from their mother's estate to the nursing home company. The carers described how Helga would use her good hand to lift her blouse, offering them the end of the tube when they came to connect it to the bag of liquid food each day. Did this represent a desire to have the food, or was it simply learned behaviour, the helpful gesture of a woman who had always been help-ful? The GP had written in his referral letter to the gastroenterology team, requesting replacement of the feeding tube, 'She seems happy enough'.

Decisions about life-prolonging treatment are made every day for those who are unable to speak for them-selves. Often these decisions are straightforward – the scales of burden and benefit are tipped so far in one dir-ection that the right course is clear. But in many other cases teams and families struggle to settle upon an answer. The ethics committee is asked to help with some of them. After a road accident or cardiac arrest, after major emergency surgery or a simple fall on an icy path, for Teddy, Pamela, Enrique, Jonathan, we gather information, listen and weigh up, consider the law and make suggestions that the medical team may or may not follow. The situation is eventually resolved: prolongation of life for one, withdrawal of life-sustaining treatment for another.

When I first wrote my advance decision to refuse treatment I know I was motivated by a concern for my own welfare. In 2016 I added an asterisk after 'meaningfully' and wrote a short addition: 'By communicate meaningfully I mean being able to convey my thoughts to my family and friends, whom I love dearly. I do not wish to have my life prolonged if I am unable to communicate with them by any means and do not have a realistic prospect of recovery to a state in which meaningful communication is possible.' The original reason for writing my advance decision then was selfish; I wanted to record my wishes clearly in a legally binding way, because I'm a participator. I answer back to the radio in the kitchen, I'm prone to making ill-informed comments on Twitter, I've always had my hand up to ask a question. I am certain that the limit of my ability to be happy would be reached once I am unable to join in. I'm not afraid so much of losing verbal fluency – communication happens in many subtle ways – but I do not want my life to be prolonged in an existence in which I am unable to convey anything of meaning to those I love, in particular being able to let them know that I am contented; that is where my own line is drawn.

However, over the years I have come to realize that my decision is not really about me. Much of the suffering in these situations is done not by the person at the centre of the decision, who in many cases is oblivious to what is going on. Rather, it is the family who carry the burden – of anxiety, anger, guilt – and they may continue to carry that heavy burden long after the central player has left the stage.

I now see that there is a second and better motivation for setting down my views explicitly. I do not want my family, ever, to be handed that burdensome decision. I don't want them to be gathered in a ward sister's office with its pinned-up thank-you letters and staffing rotas or to be walking together by the river, trying to work out whether I am conscious of their existence, and what I would wish for my future. For me, writing an advance decision is simply an act of love.

Why do my patients so rarely have a valid advance decision to refuse treatment? Those who are oldest, or who have frailty or multiple conditions, are most at risk of some life-changing event, but my experience and that of my geriatrician colleagues is that hardly any of our patients have independently made a specific plan about their future care. As with so many of the subjects of very old age that we don't discuss, the barriers are both practical and emotional. Part of the difficulty lies in not being given the knowledge that making an advance decision is an option.

I'm taken back to the antenatal classes I attended with my husband in London more than twenty years ago. We were discussing our plans for having our first-born babies. Natalie, sharp and funny, worked for HR at Marks and Spencer, and was determined to have a home birth. She'd looked around the local midwife-led unit, an annex to the big obstetric department, but she was alarmed by even that more intimate, less medicalized setting. 'I'm not having the Bean in there,' she said. 'It smells of hospital.'

I kept quiet. I liked the smell of hospital. To me hospital smelled safe, and it smelled as if you could get hold of lots of doctors quickly if you needed them. I was definitely going to have my baby in hospital.

But Natalie's decision was right for her. She had been told about the limitations of access to emergency help at a home birth, but also about the good outcomes for babies born at home to healthy mothers with uncomplicated pregnancies. The important thing about her decision was not so much what decision she made, but the fact that she had been given enough information to enable her to make it.

The next issue is that while we might be aware that making an advance decision is a possibility, it feels too complicated, too bureaucratic. Together we seem to be making this situation more difficult than it needs to be. We even get the name of the process wrong. Medical notes and the internet abound with mistaken references to *advanced* decisions, which makes the exercise sound like some sort of A level in complex moral philosophy. These are not 'advanced' decisions requiring a higher level of thought than the average citizen can manage. They are decisions made *in advance* of some future event, and they are not as intricate in practice as they might sound.

I've recently updated my own advance decision, adding details and recording my wishes in a database. I realized as I did so that I had little difficulty working my way through the online document recommended on the NHS website. Of course, it should be easy for me; I'm familiar with the scenarios presented, with the treatment options and with words like 'vegetative state' and 'minimally conscious state' and 'clinically assisted nutrition and hydration'. I know that refusing antibiotics for life-threatening infections means you would still be offered them for a painful toothache or a distressing urine infection. But these are not complicated themes. Many people understand that 'clinically assisted nutrition and hydration' means being given food and water either by drip or by tube through the nose into the stomach (nasogastric, usually temporary) or directly through the tummy wall just beneath the ribs (usually permanent). The various states of lowered consciousness speak for themselves. So, what else does someone making an advance decision need to know?

First, the name. There's no difference in practical terms between an advance decision and an advance directive (the latter is the Scottish version of the same thing; in Northern Ireland you can still make an advance decision and it holds legal weight, though under a slightly different process from that in England and Wales). Both are sometimes called a living will. Provided they are set out properly, they are legally binding.

An advance *statement* is something different entirely – it's a statement of wishes about care at the end of life (where you'd like to be, what music or words you might like to hear, the people you'd wish to have present, for example). Its requests should be honoured if possible, but it has no specific status in law. A statement is persuasive but is not legally binding.

Next, the process. An advance decision to refuse treatment can only be made in line with the terms of the Mental Capacity Act of 2005, which means that the person making the decisions must be acting for themselves and must be able to understand and weigh up each decision and to communicate their wishes (again, the legislation is subtly different but effectively equivalent in Scotland and Northern Ireland). When someone does not have that capacity a different process is needed. I talk about this in Chapter 16.

Third, the legal detail. If you are making an advance decision to refuse life-sustaining treatment, you must write in the document that you understand that refusing such treatment may shorten your life, and your decision must be signed, dated and witnessed.

Finally the practicalities. It's kind to share your advance decision with your family, and sensible to discuss it with your GP or anyone else treating you and give them a copy. Doctors can't abide by your decisions if they don't know what they are.

This summarizes the UK requirements for making a valid advance decision to refuse treatment. The same information can be found on NHS websites, which offer a link to a charity called Compassion in Dying, and on the websites of other charities, such as the Alzheimer's Society and Age UK. You can find it in information leaflets at GP surgeries and in libraries. The information is clear. For many these feel like quite straightforward decisions that can be recorded without fuss. You don't need the internet; you need a biro, a piece of paper and a witness.

Making one's views known in advance doesn't work the same way in the opposite direction. Many people, even the frailest, have no intention of refusing treatment. Rather the opposite, they would like to ensure that no treatment is withheld. However, you are not allowed to make a legally binding demand *for* a specific treatment.

I put my head round the door of David's room. I hadn't met him before, but had skimmed through his three-volume notes. David was in his late seventies and had been diagnosed with Parkinson's disease some fourteen years previously. At the onset his tremor and slow movement had responded well to treatment. Around seven years into the illness, though, things had become more complicated; his drug regime was expanded to a cocktail of different therapies designed to shore up his brain's dwindling supply of dopamine, the neurotransmitter crucial to movement. He'd been assessed for a neurosurgical procedure to implant a tiny stimulator deep in his brain, but the unlucky random presence of an aneurysmal blood vessel had put paid to that plan. His specialists had tried infusing a dopamine replacement through a tube directly into his intestine, which had worked for a while, before he began suffering dramatic light-headed episodes, his blood pressure plummeting. The infusions had to stop and the tube was removed. But David had soldiered on. The Parkinson's nurses talked to him on the phone every few months, tweaking his medications upwards to improve his movement, and putting the doses back down once they produced hallucinations. Over the years he'd stopped first hill-walking, then driving. He had moved into a bungalow. He walked with a frame; his wife shopped and cooked, paid bills, made appointments and set his tablets out five times each day. Now he'd had a fall and had broken his hip – the hip had been fixed, but David had had pneumonia and difficulty swallowing his drugs. He'd been delirious, hazily asleep most of the time since the fracture, and had lost a huge amount of weight in only a few days. The site team had arranged his transfer from the orthopaedic ward to a medical side room.

David was asleep now, his head sideways on the pillow, black hair neatly combed, his cheekbone as prominent as a streak of warpaint. His wife Sheila, with short sculpted hair, turquoise Cotton Traders piqué shirt, grey slacks and laced fabric shoes, was waiting to talk to me. She put down her book, a P. D. James, marking her place carefully with a strip of tasselled card, and shook my hand. Sheila shooed me quietly out of the room and we stood together outside the door as she spoke of her concerns: David's inability to eat, his voice being rendered inaudible by immobility of the muscles of speech, and the unravelling control of his Parkinson's disease. We agreed that he should have a nasogastric tube to give him some nutrition and to allow him to get his medicines safely. Referrals to the speech therapists and dieticians had already been made. The physios would work with him even now while he was still too weak to sit up. But I wanted to be realistic.

'Sheila,' I began, 'he's so fragile . . .'

Sheila stopped me. Her voice was soft, Scottish, firm. 'Ah, Dr Pollock, the thing you don't know about David is he's a fighter. He's always said he'll do whatever it takes to stay alive. Even if he's in a bad way, he'll want everything he can get.'

In its guidance for doctors who are caring for those who are likely to die within the next twelve months, *Treatment and Care Towards the End of Life: Good Practice in Decision-making*, the GMC addresses David's situation thus: *When planning ahead, some patients worry that they will be unreasonably denied certain treatments towards the end of their life, and so they may wish to make an advance request for those treatments. Some patients approaching the end of life want to retain as much control as possible over the treatments they receive and may want a treatment that has some prospects of prolonging their life, even if it has significant burdens and risks.*

The GMC's position on whether patients may make binding requests for future treatment was put to the test in 2005 by a courageous man, Leslie Burke. Mr Burke had a cruel degenerative brain disease, from which his brother had died, and he would inevitably lose the ability to speak for himself, though he would not lose his mental faculties. He was keen to establish that doctors should be bound not to withdraw his own tube feeding and hydration, even if his death may be imminent, once he could no longer speak. He wanted to ensure that his death would come about as a result of 'natural causes', an infection, say, rather than as a result of a medical team deciding to withdraw nutrition and hydration after judging, wrongly, his quality of life. Mr Burke won his initial case, but the GMC appealed successfully against that verdict, concerned that it could mean that doctors in other cases would be compelled to provide treatment that they knew would be of no benefit or could even be harmful. No one is allowed to insist upon treatment that is futile. However, Mr Burke's case emphasized an important principle. When doctors are making a decision about treatment for someone who lacks capacity – a decision that aims to be in the patient's best interests – they must take into account the patient's previously stated views about what indeed *would be* in his or her own best interests. The appeal judges felt that this afforded protection to Mr Burke – no one would withdraw tube feeding and hydration in order to allow his death, because he had stated that he did not consider this to be in his best interests.

The guidance goes on: *When responding to a request for future treatment, you should explore the reasons for the request and the degree of importance the patient attaches to the treatment. You should explain how decisions about the overall benefit of the treatment would be influenced by the patient's current wishes if they lose capacity . . . You should make clear that, although future decisions cannot be bound by their request for a particular treatment, their request will be given weight by those making the decision.*

Over the next few weeks David's condition worsened. His Parkinson's disease specialist, my geriatrician colleague Charlie, visited him on the ward, helping us to hone his medications and sharing some small private joke with Sheila that made her laugh. But David became unable to pee and had to have a catheter, and he developed a urine infection resistant to all antibiotics except the one that gave him miserable diarrhoea. Sheila sat by his bed, reading to him from the *Economist* and watching the feed bag run slowly into the tube in his nose. Just as he appeared to be improving, one afternoon he became suddenly clammy and his oxygen levels fell. Despite daily injections of anticoagulant, he'd had a clot on the lung, a pulmonary embolism. We started a stronger blood thinner, and his bony arms became blotched with bruises. Worse, his nasogastric tube kept playing up. He had nose bleeds and the tube troubled him; in his delirium he swept at it, dislodging its position so that it risked pouring liquid feed into his lungs rather than his stomach. The nurses replaced it and taped it down but it shifted repeatedly. In the fourth week, after David's tube had dislodged once more, Sheila met me with one of the trainee doctors at his door.

'Could he have a PEG again, like he had for the levodopa?' she asked.

We talked about it. In such a fragile state the procedure to insert a PEG tube carried real risks of infection or bleeding. David might well not survive the operation. We could ask the nutrition team for their view, although I knew they would be rightly cautious in the face of David's lingering infection and low protein levels. I worried. Sheila was speaking for David – I had no reason to doubt her word, but it was clear that she was dedicating her considerable determination and energy to David's survival, perhaps at any cost. Was our treatment becoming unreasonably burdensome for him? He had lost further weight, his confusion didn't seem to be settling, and there was no sign of any recovery of his ability to swallow. Some days I put my face close to David's when he seemed to be speaking, but I couldn't make out any words. What did he want to say? His thumbs up and down gestures were inconsistent, obscured by tremor at one moment, entirely absent the next.

I asked Charlie for his opinion – he'd known David for years.

Charlie grinned and rolled his eyes. 'Of course David

wants everything. That's how he and Sheila have always done it.' He clapped me on the back. 'See what the nutrition team say.'

Months later, a card arrived from Sheila, thanking the ward staff for their care. It ended: *The tube feeding is going well – I am a dab hand at setting it up. David is lying in his bed in the conservatory. He is happy to be home.* She had signed it neatly – *Best wishes from Sheila and 'Mr Miracle'.*

For David the key to our getting his treatment right lay in Sheila's hands; she knew exactly what he wanted. It helped too that David himself had been so unequivocal over the years and that he'd made his wishes clear to Charlie. His determination to have treatment wasn't written down, and even if it had been, would not have been binding, but knowing his views enabled us to continue when stopping might have seemed a more compassionate option. Yet had Sheila not been present, had Charlie been on leave, David's care might have been different. Surely it would have been safer for his wishes to be recorded?

Our ethics committee cases also resolved themselves one way or another. Helga's team and her family compromised. Rather than bringing her into hospital for an endoscopy, the gastroenterologists offered a modified approach, snipping the old tube off and pushing it into her stomach before sliding a new tube into its place. The technique is slightly frowned upon because there's a risk that the old piece of tube may block the bowel on its way through, but it worked for Helga, and she lived a little longer in her nursing home, succumbing to a final heart attack some months later.

Esther, inarticulate and furious, pulled out her feeding tube once again on the ward, before being returned to her care home without any tubes, and with instructions that she should be offered soft food or sips of drinks should she show signs of wanting any. I phoned the home a few weeks later and spoke to her carer Martina, whose eastern European voice was warm.

'Oh, it was lovely,' she said. 'She came home on the Thursday, and we had a big birthday bash for her on Saturday. Rachel was here, lots of music, all the staff dancing. Esther had a bit of lemonade! Then she died on Sunday morning. We all cried. It was perfect.'

And Frank, lying apparently emotionless after his stroke, his headphones streaming music into ears that might or might not be listening. Despite his elder daughter's demands, the nutrition team declined to replace his temporary nasogastric tube with a PEG, citing the high risks of such a procedure and the poor prospects for benefit. A team from a neighbouring hospital was approached for a second opinion and concurred. He was discharged to one of the rare nursing homes who will accept someone with a nasogastric tube (these tubes are notoriously risky to manage, so most care homes decline to look after people who have them). Against all expectations he lived there uneventfully for four years, dying shortly after his 101st birthday. For those four years his daughters timed their visits to avoid meeting one another. I believe that the younger will always be convinced that Frank had been condemned to an existence that he would not have wanted. The elder will remain equally certain that by fighting for continued tube feeding she won precious years of valued life for her father. Without any idea as to Frank's own opinion we shall never know which daughter was right.

So why doesn't everybody have an advance decision? Knowing you are allowed to make a decision, and knowing it might be a good idea, and knowing how to go about it, are one thing, but actually wanting to do it – that's a different matter.

There are many reasons why writing an advance decision might be easier for me than for my patients. Some people are wary of making a commitment on behalf of their future self. They observe that our views of what constitutes a worthwhile life may evolve with changing circumstances. Not everyone has the necessary degree of certainty, even obstinacy, about their own future wishes to make a binding decision, and those who do not share that confidence in the durability of their own opinion need also to be treated with respect.

There are important cultural aspects too. My friend Tess lives in the US, in Vermont, and is surprised that more people in the UK don't have clear advance decisions. She's matter of fact. 'I have to update mine every year; it's part of the requirements for my health insurance.' Conversely many people feel they should not make their own plans, preferring instead to place their future in divine hands; there's an array of opinion across members of all the world's religions as to how much control we should try to have over our lives, and I've realized over time that it's unwise to infer from someone's religious affiliation what view they will take on the subject of medical treatment.

In addition, the very oldest people with whom I work come from a generation that tends not to question their doctors. Medical decisions, they may feel, are to be made by medics; the late-twentieth-century concept of shared decision-making has been embraced by younger people, but many of my patients carry a deference to our conversations that they may need tactful encouragement to set aside.

Eric had multiple sclerosis as well as several strokes, and I had tentatively started talking about his potential future need for a feeding tube when he told me, 'I don't know how I'll feel about that until I get there.'

'Eric, the problem is you might not be able to *tell* us how you feel about it when you get there.'

I must have sounded plaintive, for Eric patted my hand comfortingly. 'Don't worry, Doctor P, I'm sure you'll cross that bridge when I come to it.'

Most importantly I'm aware that my own plans relate to an event that from here, in my fifties, seems distant – frightening maybe, but unlikely to happen any time soon. Perhaps too, there's a failure of my imagination, an emotional detachment, that allows me to contemplate these scenarios and tick them off one at a time. That's not the case for those who are very old. For my patients these possibilities are real, and may even be imminent. Acknowledging these stark futures, pinning them down in black text, physically present on a page, adding a signature: these may be steps too fearsome to take.

As I sit here looking at my dog-eared old advance decision and the snappy new version I've created on my computer, I realize that these are not decisions we can expect everyone to make sitting alone with a form and a set of guidelines, however clear and sensitive these may be. We need to proceed more gently. Making decisions about our lives and deaths, especially for those nearest to their own ending, needs a better approach. We need to be kind, and we need to talk.

*

You can find the website recommended by the NHS for explaining and making advance decisions here:
    https://compassionindying.org.uk/choose-a-way-to-make-
    an-advance-decision-living-will/

The GMC guidance about care at the end of life is here:
    https://www.gmc-uk.org/ethical-guidance/ethical-guid
    ance-for-doctors/treatment-and-care-towards-the-end-
    of-life

13. Advance Care Plans

My budgie, Olive, begins the form belonging to Raymond.

I pick up the next form. *Reg and our children.*

Another one starts *Listening to music. I like country and western.*

I smile and continue reading.

My amazing hairdo. I want to look nice every day.

I am sitting in the staffroom of a care home, reading through the plans made by residents to be followed in an emergency.

Each plan is written on a form, the county's Treatment Escalation Plan with Resuscitation Decision. There's space for a name and address sticker, and there are clear boxes to tick, for *Do Attempt Resuscitation,* or *Do Not Attempt Resuscitation,* then several more little boxes about whether or not the person should be referred to critical care (ICU, intensive care), or would like to be transferred to hospital at all, or would wish to be given intravenous antibiotics, or is *not for life-prolonging treatment, focus on quality of life.*

There are nuances. *Unclear* is an option for several of the choices, and the word 'consider' appears often. Every older patient I see in hospital has one of these documents. Sometimes my patient arrives with a form; for others it's created within a day or two of admission. The

243

resus choice is completed. Often the other parts of the form are not. Little boxes are empty, wishes unheard.

At the top of the form there's the biggest box, titled *What is important to me.* It is almost always blank. These ones, the forms that belong to each of the residents of this care home, are not blank. I pick up the next piece of paper.

What is important to me says the title, and in the box is written *Being able to put my arm around Christine.*

There are those who feel doctors should do everything, *everything*, to keep someone alive, even up to and including the most forlorn attempt at resuscitation for someone whose mind may once have been strong but is lost, and whose body is no longer able to fight; at the other extreme are people who say 'This life is not for me', and campaign with fervent dignity for the legalization of assisted dying.

I was with my new medical students, and had drawn them the life shape picture (see pages 32 and 33), like this:

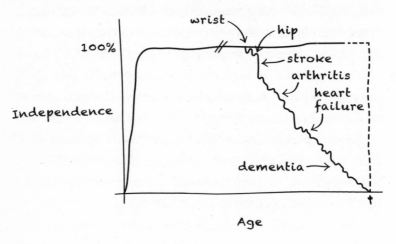

I was chivvying them to suggest ways in which the curve could be squared, so that people might live with as much independence as possible to the very end, and one of the students leaned across and took the pen from my hand and did this:

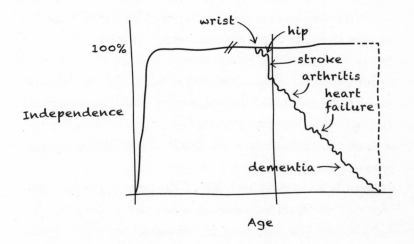

And that is a view, but it is not one I share.

Between the polarized views, in my experience, are a great many people who feel uncertain about what is the right thing to do, how much treatment is the right amount of treatment, for themselves or for someone they love. We are aware that what we think is right for ourselves may not be right for someone else, but many of us are not sure whether we can talk about it, or how, because of all the complexities of prejudice, fear and love that hamper these conversations.

*

Win is sitting by her bed, halfway down the ward on the right, and today a young woman is sitting with her, and I guess that this is her granddaughter, of whom Win is proud – she works in London, in 'media something, marketing something', Win has told me, and she studied in Paris, at INSEAD, an international business school, and she speaks several languages. The granddaughter stands as I approach. She has shiny coppery hair and a trouser suit, and she looks proudly at Win, who tells me, 'This is Marina.' Win is wearing a cream-coloured blouse and a cardigan with little roses on it, and is folding away the iPad that she and Marina have been looking at, and I draw the curtains and perch on Win's bed so we can have a talk.

Win has been in and out of hospital these past few years as her heart has faltered, and even as she sits I can see the big veins pulsing in her neck, her pretty pear-drop earrings swaying subtly, because her tricuspid valve has fallen apart, and each squeeze of her heart muscle, which should send blood forward into her lungs to be replenished with oxygen, sends a jet backwards instead, back through that leaky valve and into her right atrium and back into her veins, which flatten then distend with each beat, all wrong. And for weeks we have played around with Win's medicines and I've explained that the heart failure has made her a moving target, and twice already this year she has been admitted breathless, her lungs waterlogged, the contours of her legs obscured by swelling, and at the base of her spine a pad of fluid that can be dimpled like dough. She has needed huge doses of water tablets, diuretics, given, in fact, by injection rather than as tablets, to shift that fluid and make space in her lungs for a little air and to drive the swelling away so that her feet fit once more into her bright spotty slippers with the Velcro tabs. But another time she's been brought in dry, dehydrated, the skin of her feet wrinkled and her mouth parched, and the combination of the increased diuretics and the new drug that was meant to strengthen her heart muscle proved too much for her failing kidneys. And I've described to Win, and outline again now for Marina, how her heart failure is tricky, unpredictable, and how sometimes she'll swell like an overripe plum, full of water, but that if we overdo it with the medicines, she may shrivel up like a raisin, so we are aiming for her to be a perfect peach, and her doses will need adjusting from time to time when she's out of hospital, according to how much fluid she has on board, and Marina nods, and Win knows all that too. But there's another thing, because on this last admission Win had pneumonia too, and she almost died, and she's fallen a couple of times at home, and although her kidneys are better than they were they're not great, and she's very tired, and she's waiting now to move into a care home.

'Win?' I ask. 'Do you mind if we talk about something a bit sensitive while Marina's here?'

Win raises an eyebrow.

'Would now be a good time to have a think about

what might happen if you get unwell again when you're in the home?'

She looks sideways at Marina, who tips her head from side to side in an 'I'm OK with that if you are' way, and I go on, carefully, the path already paved because Win knows her heart can't get better, so we're able to talk about the care home she's going to. She used to visit a friend there, she likes it, and they've assured her that they have Wi-Fi, 'so I can FaceTime Marina,' for Win has mastered technology, and as well as her iPad she has a fancy phone in a glittery pink case.

I say, 'Win, I was going to fill out this form, which is about what you'd like in the future, and there's a box about what's important to you, so please may I put Marina in there?'

Win says yes, that's important, and so is having a bit of peace and quiet, so I write that down too, and Win thinks a bit and adds that she'd like to see the newspaper each week, not the national one, just a local one, 'so I can check what the Brownies are up to.'

And I explain that there are some other questions on the form, about what Win would prefer to have happen if she became very unwell, and Win puts her left elbow on the table and her chin in her hand to think about this, and I glance at Marina, who is watching her grandmother and has put her own fingers flat on her mouth, because her lips are trembling and she doesn't want Win to see. I touch Marina's elbow and say, 'Win and I have already done the resus one together,' to which Win waves her right hand dismissively to show 'none of that', and I explain that the next question is about whether she should be referred to intensive care if she was very sick. I say, 'To be honest, Win, that one's out of our hands, because I know they wouldn't want to have you in ICU, because the sort of treatments there, like being on a ventilator . . .'

I pause because Win is shooing this idea away too – move on, move on, her hand says – and I don't have to explain further that mechanical ventilation would be futile for her, that she would never come off the machine. So I say, 'The next question, Win, is quite a big one, because it's more of a decision for you than for your doctors.'

Win watches me, her chin still in her left hand, right index finger just raised, telling me she's listening, but also ready to tell me when to stop.

'Hmmmm . . . If you got really sick in the home, like if your heart got worse again or you had the sort of pneumonia you had when you came into hospital this time, the usual thing would be that they'd call an ambulance and send you in and we'd do all the stuff we do . . .'

Win puts her right hand flat on the table, while I go on.

'Blood tests and X-rays and IV medicines –' I run a finger along the back of my hand, where a drip would go – 'but some people don't want that, and they tell us they'd rather not come back into hospital, and would prefer to stay in the home and be looked after there, even if it meant they didn't get all the same treatment.'

Win takes a big breath in and lets it out slowly, and now reaches her hand out to Marina and draws her closer, so Marina pushes the bedside table out of the way and brings her chair nearer to her grandmother's and holds her hand, an old hand with a bracelet of soft gold links in a young hand with dark red polished nails. Win says, 'I've had enough of this place. I don't want to come back here. I mean, they're nice enough, don't get me wrong, Marina –' because Marina is about to say something, and Win lifts a warning finger. It's not the care she's worried about. 'I'm just tired, and if I can settle down and have a bit of rest, and stay put . . .'

I put my hand on Marina's arm, because now her lips are folded tightly together, she doesn't want to let any sound come out, and she's blinking, and I say, 'OK, Win, I can see why you've said that, and I thought that might be what you'd say after what you have been through in the last little while. Can I check if you got an infection in the home, say a cough or a urine infection or something, I'm guessing you'd like to have antibiotics if they might make you feel better?'

Win nods, a so-so, yes-and-no nod, and I continue. 'It would be just tablet antibiotics, or syrups, which might be worth a try to help you feel better, but if you got worse, and couldn't take tablets . . . well, they wouldn't be able to do the drip treatments in a care home. You'd have a choice. You could come back into hospital and we'd do our best to patch you up again, or you could stay in the home . . .'

Win wrinkles her nose. Her mind is made up. 'I don't want the hospital,' she says.

'OK,' I say. 'So, am I right, if you got super sick, like you were sick enough to *die* –' I look at her to check and she nods – 'are you saying you'd want to stay there in the home and they would look after you, even if it meant you would die there?'

'You got it,' says Win.

In Atul Gawande's Reith Lectures, delivered after the publication of *Being Mortal*, he urged those who may be coming towards the end of their life to engage with some key questions. What is your understanding of your situation? What are your fears and hopes if time is short? What are the trade-offs you are willing to make and not make? And what is the course of action that best serves this understanding?

All older people have the right to treatment, including valiant life-prolonging efforts when these are desired and stand a chance of success. My daily work, and that of my colleagues, is the provision of treatment – of antibiotics for infections, investigations for cancer, treatment for organ failure. We shore up oxygen levels, mediate extremes of blood pressure, correct a slew of metabolic upsets, stop blood leaking in one place and persuade it to flow more freely in another. But any of our patients may choose to say 'No, enough of that, I have other things to do.'

However, our autonomy is threatened the moment we become mortally unwell, when our thinking may become rapidly fogged. Most of the time that's fine. Emergency responses roll into place, ambulances are summoned, treatments are administered according to protocols designed to speed up processes and keep us alive. That is not always what we want, but unless we talk about what we want it's what we get.

'I've tried to talk to Dad about it,' Sadie tells me. 'It's hopeless. He says he knows we should talk about it, that everyone keeps telling him he should talk about it, but he doesn't want to, and I say, "It's not the sort of thing we talk about, is it?" And he says –'

Here Sadie impersonates her father, making her eyes very big and round and pulling her mouth down, and it's funny because they really are very alike. 'He says, "NOOOOOO, it is not indeed," and that's the end of the conversation.'

My friend Mike also explains, 'Mum just says, "We don't need to talk. I've made all my plans – you'll know when the time comes," and we have absolutely no idea what she's talking about, what these special plans are that she's made. I'm sure she's just fobbing us off.'

It happens the other way too, and I watch as Jeannie says, 'I don't think I'll be seeing my next birthday,' and Eloise leans in and puts her hand on Jeannie's, saying,

'Gran! Don't talk like that! You'll be fine!' but Jeannie knows she is not fine and she needs to talk about her hopes and fears, but the conversation is shut down.

It's hard to suggest ways to make these conversations easier without sounding condescending. They're easier for me partly because I'm detached – it's not my mum – but also because I'm in a position of power. I can sneak up on my patient and bring the subject into the space where we are sitting and make introductions (hello, dear Win and Marina, here is a subject you perhaps didn't want to meet, but he's here now, so let's see how we can get along), and no one is leaving until we have had the conversation.

So what helps? Perhaps it helps to know that these conversations do not always have to be detailed. It makes a huge difference if hopes and fears have been touched upon at all, if a family is able to say, 'Oh, Dad said he wouldn't ever want to be kept alive on a machine.'

Often it helps to talk about someone else's experience, how a friend was looked after, the decisions they made, so my friend Vivienne tells her family, 'Look at poor Jane, the way she is; I wouldn't want that.'

Perhaps it helps to know that conversations about future care don't always need writing down; they just need to take place, and the words drive fears away. Geriatricians see this all the time. We are often faced with a finely balanced decision, and there may be a look that passes from a daughter to her brother as she says, 'Oh, that is not what Dad would want; he's talked to us about this,' and her brother agrees, saying, 'He always said he didn't want to hang about,' and immediately a cloud lifts, and we can get his care just right, in line with what that son and daughter know of their father.

However, for many people, it is best of all to have a formal plan, detailed and documented, like Win's and like the residents of the care home where Olive the budgie lived with Raymond.

It is worth knowing some statistics. Be prepared, my reader, for they are stark. A few years ago, a research team led by Professor David Clark in Scotland collected the names of all the patients who were in hospital at midnight on the 31 March 2010 across twenty-five hospitals. The researchers excluded those who were psychiatric inpatients or were having a baby, but all the other adult patients were counted, a total of over 10,000 people. The team looked again at all the names a year later; this time they looked to see how many of the people they had counted had since died.

When I read this study the answer pulled me up short. Of all adults in hospital that one night almost 30% would not survive another year. It's not that hospitals in Scotland are bad – they're among the best in the world – or that 31 March 2010 was an especially difficult night; this research was repeated in Scotland a few years later, and in Denmark and New Zealand, with similar results. Over half of men aged over eighty-five who have been in hospital overnight will die within twelve months. Indeed, many will not survive the admission at all. The statistics are not much different for older women. A move into care is a warning flag too; only around half of those who move into a care home will still be alive a year later, not because the care is poor, but because the things that cause a move into care are also events that suggest that someone's life may be nearing its end. And there's another group of people who should be allowed to have a careful, kind conversation about their wishes, even while they are living lives that are sunny and active, and they are those who have a chronic condition. The condition is managed from day to day but the future is not discussed because no one wishes to cast a shadow, not even for a moment, and these people and those who love them are not made aware of the possibility of a sudden decline that may simultaneously present them with choices and remove their ability to choose.

The GMC advocates advance care planning, telling doctors that they should encourage discussion with anyone who has a condition that threatens their future ability to make decisions (having dementia perhaps or being at risk of a stroke or simply being very old, because things can happen suddenly). The guidance encourages conversations about 'wishes, preferences and fears' regarding future care; about what treatments might be refused and when; about 'feelings, beliefs and values'.

Here are the practicalities. First, advance care plans (unlike Advance Decisions to Refuse Treatment, ADRTs) are not legally binding. In an advance care plan we can record many things that matter: what we like to be called; whether we would prefer to sleep with a window open; whether we would like a hug or would wish to pray and with whom; whether we would rather be read Evelyn Waugh's *Scoop* or watch *Strictly*. But within a broad advance care plan, or as a stand-alone document, we may choose to make a specific plan that captures our views about what treatment we'd want – or not want – in an emergency.

Second, although they're not legally binding, a plan that covers details about our wishes for emergency care – for example, whether to go to hospital to have treatment for life-threatening sepsis – should not be overridden. Any health or care professional who does so must be prepared to justify with valid reasons the over-riding of recommendations in an advance care plan.

Third, a plan needs to be documented with crystal clarity, visible to any carers and emergency services. Advance plans are documented in different ways across the UK, and confusingly they have lots of different names. In my area we have a Treatment Escalation Plan, TEP; in other places, there's an Emergency Plan for Health Care. Many parts of the UK are adopting a scheme called ReSPECT, Recommended Summary Plan for Emergency Care and Treatment, which was developed by a collaborative team taking advice from several medical organizations but also from charities like Macmillan Cancer Support and Marie Curie, and within its processes can be heard a strong patient voice. Like my county's Treatment Escalation Plan, a ReSPECT document includes a section in which to record what is most important to its owner. The ReSPECT team explain that it '. . . creates a personalized recommendation for your clinical care in emergency situations where you are not able to make decisions or express your wishes. In an emergency, health or care professionals may have to make rapid decisions about your treatment . . . This plan empowers you to guide them on what treatments you would or would not want to be considered for, and to have recorded those treatments that could be important or those that would not work for you . . . This plan is to record your preferences and agreed realistic recommendations for emergency situations, whatever stage of life you are at.'

Fourth, it is best when making such a plan to discuss it with a nurse or doctor – a GP or a community nurse, or someone in a hospital team, who can listen, explain and ensure the plan is clear and realistic. It is possible to create a plan about emergency care for yourself without help, and there are proformas available on the internet, but a plan is much more likely to be followed if it is in a format familiar to local emergency services and is signed by a doctor or nurse deputed to do this. If your area has an agreed treatment escalation form of some sort, it's best to use it. Your GP or hospital team will be able to advise on this.

Fifth, and importantly, you are allowed to change your plan at any time and for any reason.

Lastly, in the NHS, the phrase 'advance care plan'

refers specifically to a plan made by someone who has capacity to make their own decisions. However, people who are unable to make their own healthcare decisions also deserve to have thoughtful plans made *in advance* about what would be their best care in some future emergency. The Mental Capacity Act requires that such decisions on their behalf are made in their best interests, and documents like our local Treatment Escalation Plan and the ReSPECT scheme are carefully designed so that they can be used to guide decisions that are being made on behalf of someone else.

Later, I look down the ward. Win is sitting in her high-backed chair, her head resting and her eyes closed. Marina is there too. She is bent over Win's hand, which is flat on the table, and she is painting each of Win's nails with her deep glossy red polish. As I watch, Win's eyes open for a moment and she looks down at her nails and at the smooth coppery hair of her grand-daughter. She closes her eyes again. No frown, no smile. Just ready.

Here are some of the challenges of making advance plans about what should happen in an emergency.

Sometimes it can be difficult to tell whether someone fully understands what is being discussed – whether they have capacity, in the terms of the Mental Capacity Act, to make these specific decisions about healthcare. We need to make sure they are supported and are given information in a comprehensible way. We – medical teams and families – must judge how much of the detail someone needs to understand; we must be careful not to fall into the trap of believing that someone has capacity when they make a plan that is in accordance with what we think is best for them, but questioning their capacity when they have other ideas.

Sometimes there is the question of whether family or friends are indeed benevolently motivated when they are involved in this process. I talk of 'those who love them' as if love were a given, but it is not. My geriatrician friend Connor announced indignantly, 'I wouldn't want my brother involved in any decisions for me,' and I do not think he was joking. Yet we must start somewhere, and an assumption of positive intent seems a good place to start. This is not the same as ignoring vulnerability, and we must keep our eyes open for that. If someone vehemently does not want their family to speak for them when they're unable to speak for themselves, they need to record that in advance.

Sometimes we meet those who cannot make their own decisions and who have no family, and no one who is willing or able to represent them. We may have to search out an independent mental capacity adviser, an IMCA, who will ensure that their interests are represented. This is not a speedy process, but it can and should be done.

Sometimes people do not realize the level of detail that needs to be specified, the clarity that is needed. I was listening to Heather on a train. I'd admired her coat – she was going to a sixtieth birthday party in Birmingham and I was on my way to a British Geriatrics Society conference. Heather told me about her father, increasingly fragile in a care home.

'Have you talked at all about the future?' I asked.

'Oh, he's got a DNAR,' she said firmly, and I worried, from seeing her confident look, that Heather had somehow been allowed to believe that a decision against resuscitation attempts would take care of all other future decisions too – that decisions about whether her dad would want tube feeding or treatment for life-threatening pneumonia, or indeed whether to go to hospital at all, were all wrapped up in that phrase. They are not, and nor should they be. Being 'not for resus' is not the same as being 'not for active treatment', and someone very frail who is 'not for resus' in a care home will still be taken to hospital if they become seriously unwell, and will be given lots of treatment unless plans clearly state that something different should happen.

Sometimes we have a problem with 'version control' of an advance care plan or Treatment Escalation Plan (TEP), especially when someone has been in and out of hospital. We often find that the GP's records hold a plan that is different to that on the hospital system, or that a paper version at home differs again. This is a problem across the NHS, because we have no single IT system, and this needs a central fix urgently.

Sometimes a plan is made that refuses certain

treatment, and its owner will change their mind when an emergency arises, and decide that, after all, they would like to be treated in hospital, and that's fine. They go to hospital.

Sometimes the owner of an emergency care plan has made a decision that they don't want to go to hospital, but a condition arises that, in fact, is better managed with hospital treatment; a hip fracture is the best example, because even if someone doesn't want an operation, the best way to stop a hip fracture from hurting is to screw it back together quickly, so even for someone who is very near the end of their life it's usually best to come in, have the hip fixed to ease the pain, and get back out again as quickly as possible.

Sometimes the owner of an emergency care plan is clear that they don't want ever to come to hospital, even if they are going to die, but a family or the care home staff become worried about symptoms like breathlessness, pain or agitation, and they fear that these may not be alleviated, and we need to ensure that the families are supported or staff are trained or both (remembering that in residential homes the staff are not nurses and cannot do all the things staff can do in a nursing home, and that families are not trained at all, and this may be their first encounter with death), and their GP may need to pull out many stops and call upon extra help from district nurses or from the hospice palliative care team so that symptoms can be resolved and a person's wishes can be respected, and they do not need to go to hospital.

Sometimes, and this is difficult, a family is unaware of an emergency care plan and is distressed that their relative has refused certain treatments in advance, and there are suggestions of coercion, that someone's frailty has been taken advantage of when the plan was made, and there is a humming undercurrent of painful realization that a person we love may have decided they would not like to continue being alive, would rather leave us than stay. These situations are very unhappy, especially because they usually come to light only when there is an emergency. If we are making an advance care plan, it is much, much better if we tell those who are close to us about it, and best of all if we make the plan together.

Each of the plans that I read through in that warm care home, the importance of Raymond's budgie Olive, of being able to put an arm around Christine – these are not soppy, superficial statements. They are distillations of what matters most that inform carefully structured plans made only after detailed conversations with our advance care planning nurses, who are quietly, responsively visiting one care home after another, acknowledging fears and capturing hopes. They explore and document views about resuscitation, for example, and intensive care, antibiotics and emergency admission to hospital. Any of us can ask to make an advance care plan. For those who have chronic conditions that might gradually or suddenly threaten our ability to speak for ourselves, and for those living in residential or nursing care, I believe creation of an advance care plan should be a right.

*

You can see the study by Professor Clark and his team showing the likelihood of dying among hospital patients here:
https://journals.sagepub.com/doi/10.1177/02692163145 26443

The ReSPECT documentation is described here. It is not used all over the UK, and you need to check what format is in use locally, but their website explains the principles clearly:
https://www.resus.org.uk/respect/

14. A Delicate Question

'May I ask you a delicate question?' I say.

Adeline's gaze fixes on my face.

I continue. 'Well, we've talked about the plan, that we're going to throw the book at you with antibiotics for this infection and I think you're going to get better and go home soon.' Adeline smiles. 'But . . . when you're eighty-six and have a dodgy heart too . . . well, anything can happen . . .'

I watch her expression.

'And if you suddenly keeled over with a massive heart attack or something like that, and your heart actually stopped, what automatically happens is that our team dash over and try to bring you back to life . . .'

Adeline's hand is already up. 'Oh no,' she says, 'I wouldn't want that. Just let me go.'

I squeeze her hand gently. 'I guessed you might say that, and I'm glad I asked. We'd let you go peacefully. But for now let's try to stick to plan A and get you home soon.'

Adeline and I part company. The delicate question has been answered in less than thirty seconds. Adeline is clear about what we're doing. She lives with her husband – neither still drive, but their daughter takes her shopping every week, and to church, and their son helps with bills and bits and pieces round the house. She's enjoying life, but is slowing up, and several of her friends have died. She has drawn her own line about the level of treatment she wants.

Not all of these conversations go so easily. Often I don't get past the opening line before being interrupted. Peter, for example, stops me. 'I know what you're on about – it's resus and I don't want it.' He tells me that he has had the conversation before with his GP, and is unimpressed at its being brought up again. I apologize – our recording systems are unsophisticated and hampered by a misplaced respect for confidentiality, so key information isn't readily shared between GP surgeries, hospitals and ambulance crews. People are subjected to the same questions repeatedly, and it's particularly distressing when it's something like this, a subject most of us don't want to have to think about. I amend the tag on Peter's electronic record to remind at least the next hospital team exploring his case that this is marked territory – this is his settled wish, and doesn't need going over again.

On other occasions my patient hears me out. I choose my words carefully. I have overheard some doctors ask simply 'Do you want to be resuscitated?', as if they were offering a cup of tea, and that is not fair, because resuscitation is not simple, and the outcomes of a resus attempt may not be what my patient envisages. Saying 'Do you want to be resuscitated?' makes it sound as if, provided we do it properly, resuscitation will work – the heart that has stopped beating will restart, the lungs fill with oxygen once more of their own accord. But it isn't like that, and I must be honest without being frightening. Somehow I need to explain that what is being offered is not 'resuscitation' but 'an attempt at resuscitation', and the two are very different.

I explain that unless we've made a decision the resus team will be called automatically. They'll start to press on the chest hard and will try to restart the heart electrically if the disordered heart rhythm allows (some rhythms can't be helped by shocks). Oxygen will be pushed into the lungs through a mask, then a tube will be put down into the lungs so the breathing can be done by machine. I explain that the chances of success are slim, and that sometimes we succeed in restarting the heart but the person is often not as healthy as they were before. I explain that cardiopulmonary resuscitation – CPR – 'resus' – is most likely to succeed in those who are generally well but have a sudden heart event like a bad rhythm. For those who have chronic diseases like heart failure or emphysema (COPD), the chances of surviving to be well enough to leave hospital are very small. Age alone is not a barrier to CPR, but the chances of success get slimmer.

I've had the resus conversation thousands of times now. My patients are generally over seventy-five, often over eighty-five, and usually have several things the matter at once. I've found that around two thirds are clear – they don't want resus attempts. They understand that this doesn't mean they won't be offered other treatments. Many stop me before I've finished my explanation.

Of the remaining third some want a more detailed discussion, and others want to talk things through with their family. But a few are adamant that, however slim the chance of success, a resus attempt is what they want.

Marian Willis was one of these. Tiny, wheezy and wobbly, for years she'd been batting away her family's suggestions that she might move into a care home. The duties of her faithful cleaning lady now included a weekly shop for ready meals, cigs and the *Racing Post*, and checking for any online betting wins. For over a year just swinging her legs out of bed had snatched at her breath, and after a walk from bed to bedroom door Marian would be speechless, holding the handle for a few moments before setting off again. She had come in with pneumonia and was now fighting for air. Her pulse had flipped into its distress rhythm, atrial fibrillation, and her ankles were puffy and the veins of her neck prominent, further clues that her heart was struggling, as well as her lungs. I thought the resus question would be a quick confirmation of Marian's wishes. I probably hadn't even extended my 'what's my patient feeling?' antennae. I was explaining to Marian that while we planned to treat her pneumonia and her dodgy heart, and were hoping that this would improve things, I couldn't promise success.

'Mrs Willis, I think the things we are doing will make you better, but if your heart actually stopped, I don't think we could start it again.'

She frowned at me. 'Are you talking about resus?' Words separated by breaths, wheezed through pursed lips.

'Yes . . . it's a difficult subject, but I just know that the chance of getting you back to life would be – well, so tiny.'

'I'll take it.'

'I mean, we really don't stand a chance at all.'

'I want you to try.'

I took a breath. 'I'm really sorry, Marian. We're going to try properly hard to keep you going and get you better. I really want to get you better and back home safely, but if you actually stop breathing, or if your heart stops, we wouldn't be able to start it again.'

'I want you to try.'

I was in a corner now. I needed to convey to Marian – gently, so gently – the stark reality of the situation, that with her background lung disease, and now with heart failure and pneumonia, she could not hope for a successful attempt at resuscitation. How could I allow Marian to see that I was listening to her wishes but would not be able to fulfil them? I should perhaps have backed down, given her time to gain confidence that we would do our utmost before trying to explain the limits of what we could offer, but I gave it one more go. 'Marian, I'm not really offering you a resus attempt. I'm so sorry, but it's not fair to you if I'm not realistic. I'm telling you it won't work, and it would be an awful way to go.'

'I won't care if it's awful – I'll be dead anyway.'

I was outgunned.

On the whole the resus question is surprisingly easy to discuss with very old people. Most of my patients don't want a resus attempt. Some do, and if they are usually in good health, without any major system damage, it's perfectly reasonable to be 'for resus', provided we both understand that there's a real risk of partial success, which may be a worse outcome than no success at all. As the GMC guidance puts it, *If attempted promptly, CPR has a reasonable success rate in some circumstances. Generally, however, CPR has a very low success rate and the burdens and risks of CPR include harmful side effects such as rib fracture and damage to internal organs; adverse clinical outcomes such as hypoxic brain damage* [damage due to lack of oxygen, which is often severe, affecting intellect and speech, as well as producing difficulty with movement]; *and other consequences for the patient such as increased physical disability. If the use of CPR is not successful in restarting the heart or breathing, and in restoring circulation, it may mean that the patient dies in an undignified and traumatic manner.*

With those who, like Marian, already have important chronic illnesses we can end up having an uncomfortable conversation. Some fear that being made 'not for resus' means we won't give them other treatments, that we will abandon them. However, there's a clear delineation between resuscitation attempts and other treatments, and being DNAR, Do Not Attempt Resuscitation, emphatically does not mean Do Not Attempt to Treat Me.

Some of my patients and their families have too optimistic an impression of the likely success rate. On television resus is simple – the monitor does its flat-line thing with a buzzer sounding, a handsome man in blue scrubs delivers a quick zap to the heart and, bingo, the patient wakes up and later marries him. Conveying the reality without conjuring up frightening images or destroying hope – that can be very hard.

Marian had lived with her terrible lungs for a long time – at home she didn't consider herself 'ill' – and she felt that I was denying her a chance of living a little longer. She was my courageous, determined, gritty patient, and I wanted her to feel – to know – that I was on her side. I gave her a smile and suggested that we see how things go with antibiotics, nebulisers to open up her airways and some drugs to help calm her erratic heart. I promised to come back when her sons arrived, and asked her permission to talk with them about our plans.

Her tiny knobbly hand curled into a thumbs up and she closed her eyes for a rest.

The resus chat with families needs approaching with care too. When someone's not well enough to have a proper conversation about it we turn to their relatives, and can really put our foot in it.

Vernon arrived on the stroke unit having been found unconscious by his carers that morning. His CT brain scan showed a nasty streak of clot blocking the left middle cerebral artery – the big vessel that should carry oxygen to key parts of the brain that control movement as well as the essential areas where language is both formed and understood, the brain's dictionary. We looked through his admission notes. Vernon had had a couple of mini-strokes in the past, and had become increasingly muddled over several years. He lived in sheltered accommodation, with a hot meal provided each day, and carers popped in to remind him to take his tablets and to help him wash and dress and to assist him to bed. His daughter Karen visited regularly.

Nobody knew what time Vernon's stroke had happened, so he couldn't be given clot-busting drugs (once a few hours have elapsed and the brain has been badly damaged by the stroke, the clot-busters carry a serious risk of making things worse by causing bleeding). A resus form had been completed in the Emergency Department. 'Do Not Attempt Resuscitation' was neatly ticked and signed for – but two great swipes of black biro were scored across the page, with 'Cancel' scribbled between them. A replacement form had been issued. Now the other box, 'For Cardiopulmonary Resuscitation' was ticked. Underneath, a handwritten note said 'Discussed with daughter. Wants resus'.

My registrar Nasreen and I went to see Vernon. Karen was sitting by his bed, her eyes puffy, sodden paper hankies balled in her lap. Vernon was drowsy, his right side floppy, and his eyes gazing, unmoving, to the left.

We took Karen to the ward sister's office and asked her to tell us about her dad. She sobbed. He had worked for British Telecom. He had enjoyed DIY. He had brought her up after her mum had died young. It was clear that Karen adored him. She told us how bad she felt that she worked full-time and couldn't see him as often as she felt she should – but she drove across the county twice a week to have a chat and bring him things.

'What does he like?' Nasreen asked.

'Gardening magazines,' said Karen. 'Even though he hasn't got a garden now, he still likes to look . . . and ginger nuts.'

A tiny smile, more tears. We talked about what had happened, that Vernon had had a very big stroke, and that although it was still early days it was looking unlikely that he would survive, and that if he did, he would be weaker, and that his ability to speak would not be the same as before the stroke.

Karen nodded. 'I know that. I don't want him to suffer.'

I hesitated. 'Karen, this is really sad, but I know you and the doctor downstairs had a talk about resus . . .'

Karen buried her face in her hands. 'Don't ask me about it! How can I decide? It's like asking me to turn off the switch!'

Nasreen put her arm around Karen's shoulder, while I explained.

'Karen, this is *not* your decision. You're not even allowed to make this decision. It's our decision, the medical team's decision. We are going to do everything we can to make things OK for your dad, but if he slips away, we are not going to try to bring him back, because we won't be able to. You have done all the right things, and I'm really glad you are here with him now, but you are not to carry any burden about this decision. That's our job, not yours.'

The Emergency Department doctor hadn't meant to make Karen feel that she had the responsibility for making a life-or-death decision for her father, but it's easy to let that happen by mistake. Resuscitation is not a treatment for normal dying. It does not reverse damage that has already been done. It cannot keep someone alive or restore health when essential organs like the brain have already been dealt the sort of blow that Vernon's had suffered.

I crouched in front of Karen, lifting hankies from her lap until I could find her hand and touch her fingers.

'Karen, you have done all the right things for your dad, and you love him.'

She blinked at me, and there was another tiny smile.

'And now we're going to do all the right things, and we're going to look after him, and we're not going to do something that would make it worse, and you are going to be with him now, and when the time comes – and we don't know when that is just yet – perhaps you'll be there, and you will be able to say thank you to your lovely dad, and goodbye, and you'll tell him you love him, and it's going to be peaceful.'

We must be clear what the rules are. What is the family's role in the resus decision? And, indeed, what is the patient's? First, doctors shouldn't shy away from having the conversation because they think the patient or family will be upset. If the medical team think that a cardiac arrest is a foreseeable outcome, they should talk about resus, and be kind, sensitive and honest about it, and that may mean having a conversation with someone who is younger and has a chronic condition but does not imagine themselves to be particularly sick. Discussing resus doesn't mean someone's going to have a cardiac arrest – it's an insurance policy in case they do.

Next, if the patient is able to participate in the conversation, they should be invited to do so. I get cross when doctors make very old people 'for resus' without asking them.

One of the second-year doctors, Ben, was telling me about his patient, Thomas Clark, who had an insect bite on his leg with a creeping infection that needed intravenous antibiotics. Ben had done a thorough job, taking blood cultures to look for bacteria, and checking Mr Clark's allergies before prescribing the right antibiotics. He'd ticked 'for resus' on the form, but the space where the conversation with the patient should be recorded was blank. I raised an eyebrow, and Ben said, 'I thought we only had to discuss it if we're going to make him not for resus.' Technically Ben was correct – the rules requiring discussion presently apply to DNAR orders, not to a '*for* resus' decision.

'He's really good for his age,' Ben told me. 'I think it'd be worth a try.'

We went to see Mr Clark together. He was ninety-three and twinkly, and told me he hadn't set foot in a hospital since he picked up a shrapnel injury in 1944 – he showed us the ragged scar on his abdomen. We talked about the strong antibiotics we were giving him for the infected bite, then I started the resus conversation. Mr Clark threw his wiry arms in the air and I had to catch hold of his drip to prevent it getting twitched out of his vein.

'Good grief, I'm too old for that! I don't want to come back like a cabbage – no fear!'

We left his room on good terms – he had a beautifully loud and completely incidental murmur that would do him no harm, and I promised to come back with some medical students so they could have a listen to his heart and hear about his time fighting Rommel in the desert.

Mr Clark is not alone; often I have found that it is those people who are in the best health who are most clear that they do not want an attempt at resuscitation. It's important they are given a chance to say this.

It's not always apparent whether someone really is able to participate in a resus conversation. It's a compli-cated subject, and conveying the success and failure rates can be difficult, as is describing the process of a resus attempt honestly without making it too dramatic and frightening. I have got myself in a pickle before now trying to get this right.

Freda was a smart ninety-one-year-old lady who had had a hip fracture and had come to one of our community hospitals to get back on her feet. She was hoping to return to her own home, and I recognized the address, one of a row of pretty Georgian houses in a small local town. At the time there was a big push to encourage doctors to discuss resus more openly with patients. Freda's notes were peppered with euphemisms ('short-term memory loss', 'cognitive impairment', 'poor memory') and she wasn't sure of today's date, but she was good on long-term stuff, and had told the nurses about her years living in Singapore. She was wide awake and keen to talk about plans for getting home, and anyway her daughter was visiting, so once we'd discussed the plans for pain relief, laxatives and physiotherapy, it seemed a good idea to have a chat about resus. I sat on a footstool next to Freda's high-backed wing chair, behind which stood her daughter Lynne, willowy and wearing huge dark glasses. I described the gloomy outlook for resus attempts in even the fittest person in their nineties, and was about to explain why this meant that a resus attempt would not be a realistic or kind thing for me to offer, but Freda wasn't listening.

She patted my hand. 'Oh yes, that sounds nice. What a good plan. I'd like everything.'

I was reformulating how I could gently explain to Freda that we would indeed do 'everything' that might stand a chance of success, that might restore her to that neat house, but that 'everything' should not include a resuscitation attempt that would be vigorous, even violent, and almost certainly unsuccessful. And my eye was caught by frantic movements behind her chair, where Lynne was silently grimacing, and making throat-slitting gestures.

I learned then to think more carefully about my patient's capacity to understand the conversation – and her willingness to participate fully in it. And I learned to put more thought to the presence of a worried daughter who could see that I was painting myself into a corner and was struggling to find a tactful way to indicate that I should think again. Lynne and I had a better conversation later, and she showed me the form Freda had drawn up with her GP a couple of years ago, briefly and explicitly declining resuscitation attempts. Freda herself later that afternoon had forgotten entirely who I was, and we had a cheerful conversation instead about the posy of garden flowers her daughter had brought.

When a patient can't talk about resus, or is too anxious and upset to continue when the subject is broached, then again the rules are clear: the doctor has the responsibility for making a decision, and whenever possible this should take into account the views of the patient's family or others close to the patient, not of their own wishes, but about what the patient's wishes would be. But this absolutely does not mean the family have to shoulder responsibility for the decision. We need to check with them whether they already know the patient's views; family members, like Lynne, may know that Mum or Dad has already talked this through and decided against resus. Often for our frail and very sick patients, like Vernon with his severe stroke, the responsibility lies with the doctor – we need to explain to the family that we are not offering resus because it wouldn't work. For these families doctors are often presenting an explanation of a decision already made rather than a discussion of choices.

The situation is different when it concerns someone in physically good health, who doesn't have the mental capacity to join the conversation. Here, provided the mental capacity problem isn't due to a progressive disease like dementia, resus stands more chance of being successful, and those close to the patient bring essential insight about the quality of their life, and must be allowed to help the medical team decide what is in the best interests for the person they know better than anyone else. Even then we should try not to let a family feel that the burden of decision lies with them.

Occasionally family members or friends say, 'But I have power of attorney.' Robert was worried that we were taking his decision-making role away from him, when his mum, who had severe dementia, was admitted to hospital with a constellation of other problems. We'll look at Lasting Power of Attorney (LPA) in Chapter 17, but it was very important for us to be able to reassure Robert that although his attorney role gave him the right to be involved in decisions about his mum's care, it did not allow him to make a decision in favour of resus when it was clear that such attempts would be hopeless. Having power of attorney does not mean you must be responsible for making all the decisions; attorneys need to work with medical teams to get to the right decision. In the end, offering resus is a medical decision.

So, what really are the chances of success? Am I right to be pessimistic, trying to steer many of my patients and their families away from resus attempts? A while ago I started looking at the statistics. For some years UK hospitals have been voluntarily collecting data on their resus attempts and contributing the results to the National Cardiac Arrest Audit (NCAA). The analysts study various aspects, starting with where in the hospital the arrest happened, then looking at what heart rhythm the patient was in (it's a lot easier to rescue people from a rhythm called ventricular fibrillation, where the heart is quivering and can often be shocked back into a normal beat, than it is to reverse a nasty state called Pulseless Electrical Activity, where the monitor shows a heartbeat, but there's no blood circulating). The data analysts look at whether the heart was persuaded to push blood around again, called 'restoration of spontaneous circulation', and crucially they look at whether the patient then went on to make a recovery and leave hospital – the rate of survival to discharge. When I looked at their first publication in 2014 the NCAA data suggested that the survival to discharge rate for people aged over eighty who had a cardiac or respiratory arrest in hospital was around 9%. I was surprised that almost one in ten people aged more than eighty might get well enough to leave hospital after a full-blown cardiac or respiratory arrest. I checked with our medical registrars, who are usually the senior figure at crash calls (consultants tend to be let off this duty, though we must keep our skills up to date – I have to attend an advanced lifesaving course every three years). The registrars too felt this figure didn't tally with their experience. I asked my hospital's resus team for our local data. Our 'survival to discharge' rate appeared to be in line with the national results. Then I requested the files of all those 'resus survivors'. I looked at all the detailed notes from 2012 and 2013, and over later years I was helped by junior doctors to look at those from 2014 (thank you, Hamish) and 2015–16 (thank you, Ella and Camilla).

The notes made sobering reading. Several of those who were recorded as having had a successful outcome hadn't had a cardiac arrest at all, nor had their breathing stopped. Rather, in one case the patient had had a seizure, but the 'crash team' had been called by an inexperienced nurse. In another a frail man had several episodes during which he lost consciousness because his blood pressure dropped very low when he stood up – simply putting him flat on the bed restored his pulse. Two women had had 'funny turns', becoming pale and pulseless, but had recovered spontaneously by the time the resus team arrived. One patient hadn't had attention from the team at all; his hospital number had been included through an administrative error. One by one we had to exclude supposed success stories, and the number of patients who had truly survived a resuscitation attempt dropped.

However, there were some survivors. Each year we found two or three who had genuinely done well – perhaps 4 or 5% of those who had had resus attempts. Each conformed to a pattern; they were active people over the age of eighty who had had very few illnesses. They came in with a heart problem – a heart attack or a dodgy heart rhythm. None of the 'good' survivors had pneumonia or other lung problems, or strokes or dementia. None had a surgical problem like peritonitis or a hip fracture. Each of those who survived to go back to their own home had come in with just one condition, affecting only their heart, and had a cardiac arrest either in the Emergency Department or in one of the cardiology wards. Each of them had a short but essential visit from the resus team and was shocked back into a normal rhythm quickly. Some then went off to the cardiac catheter lab, where the cardiology team injected dye to identify the furred-up heart artery, and opened it using impressive manoeuvres with tiny balloons and stents. Clinic letters afterwards testified to the positive outcomes: 'It was good to hear that John is playing golf again', 'Mrs Marks was pleased to be told that she is allowed to resume driving'.

In some years there were one or two people who also 'survived to discharge' after a stormier admission that included a full-blown resus attempt. Their stories were difficult to read, as 'survival to discharge' did not mean they had made a good recovery. Instead they had been discharged to a nursing home where they had died a few weeks or months later, or they had gone home but were persistently confused and needed round-the-clock care provided by their families; these seemed sad endings. Strikingly when resus was discussed again with these patients or their families no one opted for another attempt. I suspect that, should the data in the national audit be subjected to the same level of scrutiny, results from other hospitals would be similar.

We try to keep our resus conversations as kind but as honest as possible, but when we bump into someone like diminutive Marian, clinging on to life and the racing tips, desperately ill, we must tread a careful path. Marian looked as if she may well be going to die and I didn't want her to be frightened. I was sure that whatever I said she would believe that being made not for resus would mean we'd given up on her. My priority was not to let her feel abandoned, but I wasn't going to lie to her either.

The GMC offers some advice for situations like Marian's, when resus attempts will not be successful and we are trying to work out how to explain this. *You should not withhold information simply because conveying it is difficult or uncomfortable for you or the healthcare team.*

Oh, Marian. I could cope with the difficulty and

discomfort of telling you that resus should not be offered. It was not me that I was worried about.

Later that evening, I met her sons. Tall, broad-shouldered men, they shared a smile with one another when I described the resus discussion Marian and I had had.

'Oh, that's Mum all over,' said the elder.

'She does her own thing,' the younger added, pulling his jaw sideways, showing me the awkwardness of his mum's 'own thing'. 'Stubborn . . .'

His brother joined in. 'Bloody-minded . . . She wants to go on for ever, but we know she can't.'

Marian's sons were realistic. We talked through the treatment she was having, all the things that were giving her a chance of survival, and we talked about resus, and the younger son shook his head. 'I've seen it – chap at work collapsed, the paramedics came, working on him.' He paused, shivered and screwed up his face. 'It's not the way she'd want to go, if she knew.'

Cardiopulmonary resuscitation is not a treatment for ordinary dying. It has become iconic, emblematic of life, death and twenty-first-century medicine. For many it's perceived as an affront, an unwanted barrier to a natural and dignified death. For a few it's a moment of rescue, a lifeline that catches them as they fall, down, down, and swings them back onto solid ground. For others it seems to represent a gateway to a life that might continue just as it is now, unchanged, unchallenged, but that gateway is a mirage, illusory.

I walked with her sons towards Marian's room. She lay, the nebuliser mask almost covering her eyes, and the stream of air escaping round the mask blew her fine hair around her face like dandelion fluff. We would have a conversation, a careful, calm, gentle conversation that would touch upon understanding, hopes and fears, and which would in the end bring us to the answer to a delicate question.

*

You can read more about CPR and resuscitation decisions at the website of the UK Resuscitation Council here:

https://www.resus.org.uk/faqs/faqs-dnacpr/

15. 'I Know You've Got to Do It'

Three years ago, a GP trainee, Will, and I were about to see Albert. He was eighty-six and had just arrived in hospital from a nursing home where he had become increasingly yellow over the last few days. He was sleeping right now, curled up in a bed by the window. His right arm stretched across his body, long and thin, tattooed and bruised. Between pillow and sheet a tuft of wiry hair and an angular cheekbone were all that I could see of his face, and his hip lifted the light blanket into a sharp triangle.

Will and I had looked through Albert's summaries on the computer system. Albert had been admitted a couple of times the previous year, then he was in hospital again from mid-September until just before Christmas, when he was discharged to a nursing home. I noticed the address: a big new home that specializes in the care of those with the most severe dementia. Albert had only been there a few weeks and now he was back.

Albert's problem list was long, and was in medical shorthand: *T2DM, IHD, HTN, CCF, AF, PVD, CKD, OA.* Type 2 diabetes mellitus, ischaemic heart disease, hypertension, congestive cardiac failure, atrial fibrillation, peripheral vascular disease, chronic kidney disease, osteoarthritis. These were his background problems, the ones he'd been living with for years. They're common and often coexist.

The summary went on. *Admitted with AKI* [acute kidney injury]. *Treated for HAP* [hospital acquired pneumonia]. *Delirium, dementia. Developed anaemia, transfused two units. Leg ulcers reviewed by vascular team, no surgical intervention.*

It ended: *Patient and family kept fully informed throughout.*

Will and I looked behind us to where Albert was folded into the bed. He was still asleep, a bag of saline running drop by slow drop into a vein.

We turned back to the screen and called up Albert's blood results. His creatinine, a marker of kidney function, was well off the scale. I wondered what it usually was – whether this was a change from Albert's baseline. I clicked on an icon that would show me his previous results. The screen became crowded with numbers. That was page 1. I clicked to page 2. The same. Page 3. More. Screen after screen of blood results.

My palms had gone sweaty and I screwed up my eyes, angry prickles making me blink. Will counted the results. Between 19 September and mid-December Albert had had seventy-seven blood tests. Almost every day during his last hospital stay – seventy-seven times – someone had approached him, rolled up his sleeve and taken a couple of phials of blood. Each time his creatinine had been measured, together with his salts – sodium and potassium. Often they'd checked his full blood count too – measurements of his haemoglobin level and how many white cells he had for fighting infection, and the platelets that would help his blood to clot. They'd requested CRPs (C-reactive protein) testing for inflammation. Albert's CRP was always a bit high, which didn't signify anything in particular. His sodium and potassium occasionally strayed just outside the normal boundaries. His white cell count bobbed up and down a bit. He became anaemic and was given a blood transfusion. His creatinine was terrible every time it was checked, because it was never going to get any better.

Albert's old notes arrived. We traced his passage through the hospital: a few days on the acute medical unit in September, then a transfer to a cardiology ward. Later, he was shunted from cardiology to their 'buddy' ward, which is one that specializes in head and neck surgery. The medical division is always bursting its seams and has to move its patients into surgical beds, and our head and neck ward takes the overflow when the cardiology ward needs space for a new patient. Albert stayed a couple of weeks on 'head and neck' before moving to a rehab ward, and for a few days it looked as if things might improve. Then his leg ulcers got bad again and he was moved on to a care of the elderly ward, where in the end it was acknowledged that Albert wasn't going to be able to return to residential care and plans were made for his move into the nursing home.

Throughout his notes there was such careful stuff – concerns about his water tablet doses, which were adjusted several times; notes regarding his poor nutrition, and a referral to the dieticians, who recommended supplements; there was a worry that he may be developing a bony infection, osteomyelitis, under one of his leg ulcers. He had three chest X-rays and there was talk of a CT scan to look for a clot on the lung – that scan couldn't be done because his bad kidneys would be further damaged by the dye involved – but there was an MRI to check for the osteomyelitis. Physiotherapists documented Albert's reluctance to participate in therapy, and nurses noted his confusion and restless nights. Albert's blood sugar levels had been checked by a finger-prick blood test four times a day, every day, for three months.

Among the paperwork that had come in with Albert from his nursing home was the Treatment Escalation Plan that had been created during his last admission. His 'not for resus' status was clear, but beneath that the directions for those looking after him were equivocal. A box was ticked: *consider hospital transfer*; and another: *may be for life-prolonging treatment*.

At the top there was the blank area: 'What is important to me'.

I stepped back from the paperwork for a moment and found my hands were curling and stretching, as if trying to shake something off that had stuck to my palms.

Late that afternoon, Albert's son and daughter arrived and sat on brown plastic chairs next to Albert's bed. Will and I talked with Paul and Jan, and heard how difficult the autumn had been for all of them.

'Not being funny,' said Jan, 'I mean, the care is

amazing . . . but Dad hates hospitals. He wouldn't even visit Mum when she was in here.'

Paul had come straight from his work in a builder's merchants, and looked tired.

'Your dad had a lot of tests last time,' I said.

Paul looked uncomfortable. He crossed his legs and stared down at his heavy boots. 'Yeah, well . . . I know you've got to do it.'

Albert's son Paul articulated one of the difficulties that patients and families face. There's a perception that whatever the medical team are doing, it's for the best. There are vague notions about the Hippocratic oath, about the sanctity of life, the duties of a doctor. However, many of the tests and treatments offered towards the end of a long life are not clear-cut in their benefit. How do doctors decide what they've 'got to do'?

The Hippocratic oath is not taken by many doctors these days; it's sworn at graduation ceremonies in some medical schools around the world, but other schools use a modified version, or a different oath entirely, or none. Some of the Hippocratic exhortations have stood the test of time: to act for the benefit of patients, to respect confidentiality, to avoid actions that are 'deleterious or mischievous', but other parts of the oath are anachronistic. It includes invocation of support from the gods Apollo and Aesculapius and various other gods and goddesses.

In the UK the duties of a doctor are laid out by the

GMC. The GMC issues our licences, and decides whether we are fit to practise, and can strike doctors off its register – practising without a GMC licence is illegal. The GMC sets the standards by which doctors are judged and provides a firm description of those standards. The GMC's ethical advice is issued in the form of guidance, but it would be an unwise doctor who chose to ignore that advice, which is considered, detailed and aligns with the law.

In the GMC document *Treatment and Care Towards the End of Life*, there is guidance that says *Decisions concerning potentially life-prolonging treatment must not be motivated by a desire to bring about the patient's death, and must start from a presumption in favour of prolonging life. This presumption will normally require you to take all reasonable steps to prolong a patient's life.*

That statement feels good and safe, and is clear about the duties of care. But too often it feels as if that's where our collective understanding of the situation finishes. We must read the next sentence. The same guidance continues: *However, there is no absolute obligation to prolong life irrespective of the consequences for the patient, and irrespective of the patient's views, if they are known or can be found out.*

Some treatments may present more of a burden to the patient than may be acceptable to them. People's views are individual, and should be both discovered and respected. The three great barriers that I described at the start of the book, prejudice, fear and love, already stand in the way of conversations about what treatment is right for those who are coming towards the end of a long life, and now we've added another barrier, confusion. It's worth being completely clear. When we are making plans with or for someone about their care, and those plans include decisions not to use certain life-prolonging treatments, we are not talking about euthanasia, which is killing people and is illegal in the UK, nor about assisted suicide or assisted dying, which is deliberately helping someone to kill themselves and also illegal. We are talking about conversations that allow medical teams to understand our wishes and beliefs, that enlighten those who care for us so that we can decide together what treatments would be of overall benefit to us. That may include deciding against certain treatments.

Here I should lay out my view. I believe that many people suffer for both physical and existential reasons, and although I believe that good palliative care should be available to all, I know that it does not – cannot – always relieve suffering. I do not dismiss that suffering; however, I also believe that it is impossible to legislate to allow assisted dying in a way that protects vulnerable people. I believe that many older people, for reasons to do with the way our society is structured, can be made to feel worthless and burdensome. I believe that there is inherent value in imperfect lives, that when one looks beyond the surface, beyond the physical and material on which so much is judged, no life is, in fact, perfect. I believe that it is too easy for someone whose life may be judged worthless and imperfect by others to be made to judge themselves that way too – to be made to feel so worthless and imperfect that they would be better off killing themselves or opting to be killed. I believe that is wrong.

However, the debate about assisted dying, which remains illegal, has distracted us from a more pressing need. We need to talk more openly and kindly about the benefits and limitations of treatment in those coming towards the natural end of a long life – about *unassisted* dying, but also about making the most of limited time, about living well to the end.

It's one thing talking about our own wishes. Speaking for someone else may feel more difficult. Albert's discharge summary stated *Patient and family kept fully informed throughout*, which is a standard phrase but does not ring quite true. Albert himself was in a state of sleepy or agitated confusion throughout his previous admission. How can Albert have been 'fully informed'? And Paul and Jan may have been informed about Albert's tests and treatments, but there's a sensation that something was missing, which is their active involvement.

Again, GMC advice is clear. When deciding about treatment for someone who is unable to make their own decisions, at any stage of life, doctors must consider the *views of people close to the patient on the patient's preferences, feelings, beliefs and values, and whether they consider the proposed treatment to be in the patient's best interests.*

There's a balance. It's important that Paul and Jan don't feel they are made responsible for medical decisions.

Neither have legal proxy status, such as LPA. But that doesn't matter – being a legal proxy gives someone the right to *make* a decision for someone else, and without it the decision-making rests instead with the doctor. But families and friends without power of attorney are still part of the process of decision-making. Paul and Jan's views count because they know their dad – they have dropped everything to be with him here, have asked a colleague to cover a shift, will push coins into the maw of the car park ticket machine, or will wait later in the dank February drizzle for the bus back home.

Just as the public debate about assisted dying has stopped us talking freely about unassisted dying, the introduction of LPA status has muddied the waters about the involvement of families in decisions. Sometimes families fear they cannot speak because they don't have formal power of attorney or legal proxy status. Even worse, sometimes families are led to believe that their view doesn't count because they don't have this official status. That is nonsense.

It's not easy. Paul and Jan knew little during that previous long admission about Albert's medical conditions and the pros and cons of various tests – why should they? And when I was looking back through Albert's notes I was using the high-minded doctor's favourite instrument, the retrospectoscope, which allows us to pour scorn in hindsight on the decisions of our predecessors, who were acting in good faith. But medicine runs so fast now – protocols drive decisions, and the blood sugar record demands that checks are done frequently until Albert's sugars are consistently below eleven for three days in a row, which they never are, nor should they be; and the protocol for managing heart failure demands 'daily U and Es' – tests of kidney function and salt levels – and his doctors no longer have to wonder whether to do each test, making each request individually, but rather can click one button that generates automatic requests, so Albert gets a test of his kidney function every single day until someone thinks to cancel the order. It's hard to find a moment to pause and look at the whole picture and consider whether what we are doing is consistent with someone's 'preferences, feelings, beliefs and values', especially when they can't tell us what these are. Yet it's essential we do this and are given time to do this. We need to spend more time doing something right now, in order to spend less time doing things that are wrong later.

Will and I took Jan and Paul to the end of the ward. That's another problem, finding enough space in which to talk privately, but we drew the plastic chairs into a little circle, and pretended no one could hear as people banged through the double doors beside us. We talked briefly about Albert's life – he was a farmhand, then did security work, night watchman. His wife Amy died a while back.

'He was a bit lost without Mum,' said Jan, and Paul rubbed the back of his neck, still looking at his boots.

Jan explained how the house got into a state and Albert had moved into a residential home. 'But he never settled really; he didn't like it.'

'What did he miss about home, apart from your mum?' I asked.

'Oh, going out,' said Jan. 'He was always a walker; he would walk round the edge of town, off in the fields, but he'd not been able to for a while even when he was at home, because of the heart and that . . .'

Paul uncrossed his legs. 'Outdoors, that's what he liked.'

We talked about Albert's medical situation. I explained that I thought previous teams had done everything they could to make him better. They had looked for reversible things, but many of his problems were not going to go away. And now he was yellow, which suggested that something had gone wrong with his liver too; he had no abdominal pain and, looking at the pattern of his blood results, this yellow jaundice was most likely due to a blockage, probably a tumour, although it could be something else. I explained that a scan had already been booked by the team who saw Albert last night. Paul leaned forward and looked at the floor. Jan's right hand was a fist in front of her mouth. I went on. 'I'm not sure that's what your dad would have wanted.'

Jan and Paul looked up.

'I wonder, did your dad ever say anything about what sort of treatment he'd want, if he got ill?'

They glanced at one another and shook their heads,

and Jan said, 'It's not the sort of thing you talk about, is it?'

They both looked down again, and their shoulders sagged with the burden of not knowing.

I thought back to a technique I was taught by my wise colleague Peter, and explained, 'Even though it's not something you've talked about, we could think about it like this: if your dad was here with us, and he was not so poorly – say he was the way he was a few years ago – what would he say about the man in the bed in the situation he's in now?'

Paul straightened up and put his wide hands, which were covered in scrapes and scars, on his knees, and said, 'He'd say no. He'd say let that fellow go. Let him have a bit of peace.'

Jan looked at Paul and said, 'You're right, Paul, that is what he'd say.'

Everything fell into place. We didn't have to do that scan. It might have shown something technically treat-able, a stone that might be fished out or a little tumour in a critical place that could be bypassed by a stent, but putting Albert through scans and treatments wouldn't change the rest of his illnesses. I explained that if we found a treatable cause for the jaundice, we might extend Albert's life, but most likely only by a little, as his other illnesses meant he was likely to die fairly soon. I couldn't be sure when; it might be days or weeks, or even maybe months. Investigating and treating the jaundice would mean he'd have to stay in hospital, at least for a few days, and in any case the scan might well show something completely untreatable. The jaundice didn't seem to be bothering Albert. Paul looked back up the ward to where his father lay in the far bed by the window.

'It's not what he'd want. What is it they say, quality not quantity? That's where we're at, I reckon.'

We talked about Albert's tablets. Would it be a good idea to cut them down, stop ones that weren't making him feel better?

Jan smiled and said, 'Dad never liked tablets. And some of the staff got upset with him if he wouldn't take them.'

We would stop checking Albert's sugar levels unless he was overly thirsty. In fact, we'd plan no more blood tests at all. What would make Dad a bit happier? I wondered. Might he like a half-pint of something – cider? Beer?

Now Paul grinned. 'Would he!'

What else? Did Dad enjoy watching the TV?

'He liked watching the football,' Paul told us. 'But he wouldn't have a clue who's playing now.'

That evening Albert went back to the nursing home. The manager had been phoned and would get a copy of his discharge summary and escalation plan, both of which would also go to his GP. We didn't know when Albert was going to die, but if – when – he got sicker in the home, they would not send him back to hospital.

A few months after meeting Albert, I saw Jan again, queuing to pay in Tesco. I'm hopeless at recognizing patients and families when I meet them in a different context and was struggling to work out where I'd seen Jan before when she told me.

'We saw you with Dad. Albert Lester. He was in Beech House. He went on a couple of weeks back.'

'Oh, Jan, I'm sorry. How was it?'

Jan put her basket on the checkout shelf and swept her hands down the front of her coat.

'Do you know, doctor, it was fine. He looked a bit better at the start to be fair. We took him for a spin in Paul's car, up to the beacon. And Paul sat with him back along and watched the football, and they had a pint. Well, Paul did anyway. I don't think Dad had more than a sip. And then I saw him the Sunday and he looked a bit peaky, but they didn't call the ambulance, just settled him down, and the next day the home rang and said he was gone . . .'

Jan looked away from me, sideways and upwards. Her lips pressed together hard for a moment, and she was squeezing the fingers of one hand with the other. She screwed her eyes up, then opened them and went on. 'A relief really . . . I know you shouldn't say it, but it was, for him, so there you go.'

When someone cannot make important healthcare decisions for themselves, and no attorney has been appointed, these decisions rest with the doctor leading the medical team. It is unusual for our patients to have appointed an LPA for health and care, and when there is no such legal proxy GMC guidance reiterates that the doctor must *seek information about the patient's circumstances; and seek views about the patient's wishes, preferences, feelings, beliefs and values. The doctor may also explore which options those consulted might see as providing overall benefit for the patient, but must not give them the impression they are being asked to make the decision. The doctor must take the views of those consulted into account* . . .

The GMC's guidance marches hand in hand with the law as expressed in the Mental Capacity Act, and as well as emphasizing the necessity to act in the patient's best interests, the guidance requires doctors to consider which options for treatment would provide overall clinical benefit for the patient. It also requires us to consider *which option, including the option not to treat, would be least restrictive of the patient's future choices.*

And whenever I read this guidance I turn things over in my mind, because being dead is a pretty restrictive option in terms of future choices. But Albert's choices were limited already, both future and indeed present, and further treatment for Albert represented a more restricted future than the 'bit of peace' Paul had suggested he'd prefer.

I hope that my geriatrician colleagues will forgive me for describing this process, because it is only a part of our job, and the majority of our work involves active treatment, even some heroic snatching from the jaws of death, the pursuit of recovery, restoration of health, and perhaps a great deal more laughter than you might guess. We often have long-term relationships with our patients in outpatient clinics as we work together to manage complex chronic conditions like Parkinson's disease or heart failure. It's not all about the ending. But this is an important part of our work, finding out our patients' 'wishes, preferences, feelings, beliefs and values'.

Paul and Jan must not be asked what *they* want for their dad; they are being asked what he would have wanted. When our patient is unable to speak for himself those who know and love him should be invited to step in, and must be allowed to speak and be heard.

*

You can find the GMC's guidance for doctors about capacity and consent here:
https://www.gmc-uk.org/ethical-guidance/ethical-guid ance-for-doctors/consent

And about treatment towards the end of life here:
https://www.gmc-uk.org/ethical-guidance/ethical-guid ance-for-doctors/treatment-and-care-towards-the-end-of-life
https://www.gmc-uk.org/ethical-guidance/ethical-guid ance-for-doctors/consent

16. Capacity

Lillian calls me over. 'I want to see the doctor.'

'Mrs Jason, it's nice to meet you. My name is Lucy Pollock. I am one of the doctors.'

'I know who you are. But I don't want to see you with your –' she casts a withering look over me, assessing my earrings, dress, shoes – 'silly ways.'

Lillian has a florid bruise cupping her left cheek and chin. Above her right eye, three greying Steri-Strips maintain an uncertain grip over a scabby laceration. There's another older bruise over her collarbone, and peeping out from her NHS pyjama sleeves I can see the pink and purple scars of burns that are only slowly healing. Her hair sticks up stiffly from her head, two-tone; it's grey for the first inch and a half, but the next inch is brown. Lillian has her cardigan on over her pyjamas and has pulled her greasy coat from the bedside locker. She is poised for flight, away from me, away from the ward, back home and safely into the past.

'I'm sorry about that, Lillian. I'll try not to be silly. How can I help?'

'I want to go home. I want to go home now.'

She thumps the bedside table with her fist and tea sloshes out of her cup.

'Why can't I go home? I want to go now.' Her voice has risen, and she shouts close to my face. 'I'm going home this minute!'

I grab a towel and mop the tea.

'I'm sorry you are having such a difficult time. It must be very frustrating . . . Lillian, I know this sounds like a daft question, but do you know where we are now?'

Lillian looks affronted. 'Yes, and it's . . . it's a place . . . it's a horrible place. And I am going home.'

I promise Lillian that I will do what I can ('They all say that.') and retreat to the office, where I phone the warden of the sheltered accommodation where Lillian lives, while looking up her discharge summaries. She's had eight admissions in as many months, with falls and seizures and infections. There are concerns about her well-being and comments that 'Mrs Jason was keen to return to her own home, so has been discharged with community support'.

The warden, Robbie, is friendly. 'Oh, Lil,' he says. 'I'm sorry she's with you again. I think we've reached the end of the road here.'

'Have you known her long?' I ask him.

'She was here when I started. Five years maybe? She's one of a kind. Her neighbour used to do her shopping, though there wasn't much on the list. Tio Pepe sherry, Laphroaig whisky and Ferrero Rocher.'

Oh, dear Lil.

Robbie continues, explaining that Lil's been off the drink for several years now, but other problems have arisen. He paints a picture for me of Lillian's flat, her stressed carers, the ambulance parked outside.

'You'd think the crew lived here,' says Robbie.

Next, I look at the electronic records stored by the community trust – having access to those is a rare bonus because I work for the hospital trust, and despite the fact that both organizations are called 'trust' there seems to be no trust when it comes to sharing information. The NHS is not a seamless monolithic organization; it has management structures that maintain separation between services provided in the community and those delivered in the hospital, and too often it keeps the activities provided by both hospital and community services hidden from the staff of a GP's surgery, including the GP, and, of course, those responsible for delivering social care are kept nicely in the dark by everyone else. Thus all the memory clinic letters, the community therapists' notes and the district nurses' comments about Lillian's safety at home are hidden from most of the doctors in the acute hospital and from the GP. And even when you are granted access it's a clunky system and you need to know secret passageways to find the golden facts.

The signs started a few years ago for Lillian when she had a fall. A visit to the Emergency Department for stitches prompted an assessment by the community therapy team, and words like 'unkempt' and 'cluttered' feature in the therapist's notes. There is a comment about mouldy food in the fridge. Lillian was offered help with her shopping, which she declined; she refused to move some of the rugs over which the therapist thought she might trip. A couple of years later phone calls from a worried Robbie, after finding her outside in her nightie 'off to Dundee', caused her GP to refer Lillian to the memory clinic. Lillian didn't attend. There's a record of a visit from a community psychiatric nurse – Lillian sent her packing, angry that she'd been referred to the memory clinic when 'my memory is better than yours'. The clinic's admin team added a note explaining that as she had 'refused to engage' she'd been discharged from the memory service.

More recently Lillian's behaviour has moved up a notch. Admissions to the big hospital have been followed by spells in two different community hospitals, having further assessments and physiotherapy. Each time Lillian maintains that she is doing well at home and will not consider any other option. Carers have been sent in – initially twice daily, then thrice. The therapists have unplugged her cooker for safety. After a hip fracture a few months ago, her niece Neoma arranged a live-in carer, who slept on a fold-up bed in the living room and lasted less than a week before Lillian threw her out, outraged by the invasion of her privacy. The therapists have visited again. This time their words are more strident: 'unsafe', 'hazardous', even 'squalid'. A carer who tried to move some of Lillian's half-empty soup tins was hit with a broom.

I read on through Lillian's community notes made in

the week or two before her current admission. A district nurse has visited. She writes *Mrs J was clear about her wish to remain in her own home. Although she lacks insight into the situation, I think she has capacity.*

I wrinkle my nose.

Ah, capacity. The Mental Capacity Act 2005 sits silently on the geriatrician's shoulder on every ward round. Does Lillian have the capacity to make her own decisions about where she should live? And if not, what should we do next?

Shortly after the introduction of the Mental Capacity Act I listened to a remarkable nurse as she gave a lecture to attendees at a British Geriatrics Society meeting, and I wish I could remember her name, because I bow down before her masterly explanation of the legislation. I'll call her . . . Sister Lucid.

At the conference Sister Lucid held up her left hand to illustrate the five principles of the Mental Capacity Act. She put up her thumb and waved it at us.

'Everything OK?' she asked, and her audience nodded obediently.

She went on. 'Everything is indeed OK. The Act says "a person must be assumed to have capacity unless it is established that he lacks capacity". The code of practice reminds us that every adult has the right to make their own decisions, unless there is proof that they lack the capacity to make a particular decision. And this is the number-*one* principle –' she waved her thumb again – 'so we can also remind ourselves that someone may have capacity for *one* decision, but not for another. Thumbs up!'

Sister Lucid turned away from her audience for a moment, then whipped back round, pointing her index finger at us. 'What have *you done*?' she asked fiercely, and we wriggled anxiously. She jabbed her finger at us and asked again, 'What have you done to help that person have capacity?'

And thus Sister Lucid delineated the second principle, which is that 'a person is not to be treated as unable to make a decision unless all practicable steps to help him to do so have been taken without success'. That may be something as simple and essential as changing the batteries in a hearing aid (which incidentally don't last more than two weeks, or less if the hatch isn't opened when they're not in use). It may mean providing written information, or a translator, or treating delirium or psychosis so that a person's mind becomes clear, or providing a light-writer for a man with locked-in syndrome to operate with his eye movements. There are many ways in which to help someone have capacity.

Sister Lucid next said, 'Excuse me,' and beamed as she held up her middle finger alone, giving the bird to 200 doctors. 'You are permitted to disrespect authority figures.'

The third principle of the Act is that 'a person is not to be treated as unable to make a decision merely because he makes an unwise decision'. We are all allowed to make unwise decisions – and, oh my, how well we exercise that right! We order a juice blender, shave off an eyebrow, have an affair or invest in a glittering scheme; we make variably daft decisions every day without anyone questioning our right to do so. This works because our capacity for making these decisions is assumed to be present – we may not be sensible, but we know what we're doing. The Act's code of practice reiterates that 'everybody has their own values, beliefs, preferences and attitudes', and goes on to say 'a person should not be assumed to lack the capacity to make a decision just because other people think their decision is unwise. This applies even if family members, friends or healthcare or social care staff are unhappy with a decision'.

Sister Lucid went on. She pointed to the wedding ring on her fourth finger and rolled her eyes as she said, 'It was the *best* day of my life, according to my husband,' and she reminded us that the fourth principle is the '*best interests*' clause. The Mental Capacity Act formalized the common-law principle that an act done, or decision made, on behalf of a person who lacks capacity must be done, or made, in his best interests. It is to this core fourth principle that the courts will turn should they need to review acts done by an attorney, or a medical or social care team. If a dispute arises, the pivotal question will often be whether the attorney or other decision maker was acting in the person's best interests.

Finally she waved her little finger at us. 'My little

finger, the *least* finger, tells us the fifth principle. This is that we should look as hard as possible at all the options, to try to find the one that is least restrictive. We must always question if we can do something else that would interfere less with the person's basic rights and freedoms.'

So, those are the five principles illustrated by Sister Lucid's five fingers. The rules of our society are largely based on ancient Greek philosophy, the pillars of Aristotelian ethical thinking – beneficence (doing good), non-maleficence (doing no harm), justice and autonomy. And, among these, autonomy towers. Respect for the rights of the individual; it's what gives us a vote and freedom of speech, and it protects us from being unfairly locked up. And that includes being moved into a care home against our wishes.

How do we know whether Lillian has capacity at all to decide whether she should continue to live in her own home?

The Mental Capacity Act holds that someone lacks capacity if they *not only* have an impairment or disturbance that affects the way their mind or brain works, *but also* that the impairment or disturbance means that they are unable to make a specific decision at the time it needs to be made. We must apply this 'two-stage test' to Lillian's situation.

First, does Lillian have an impairment of or a disturbance in the functioning of her mind or brain? And then, second, does that impairment mean that she is unable to make a specific decision (in this case about continuing to live in her own home) at the time when she needs to make that decision?

And the answer to the first part is 100% yes. Lillian has dementia. The disintegration over several years of her memory, orientation, planning – this is well beyond eccentricity. She's had enough tests and scans for us to know that there's nothing reversible here. The only reason Lillian does not yet have a formal diagnosis is that she refused to see any member of the dementia team – she simply refused to be given a diagnosis of dementia, but she has it.

Having dementia does not of itself mean Lillian lacks capacity. Someone who has dementia may still be able to understand decisions about their care, weigh up their options and come to a decision, with support from their families, staff or both. Many others who have dementia or similar conditions may have capacity for some decisions – toast or cereal, which radio station – but do not have capacity, even with support, to make specific healthcare decisions. Decisions must be seen as both time and subject matter specific. Someone may not have capacity in the evening, the traditional 'sundowning' time when those with dementia tend to become more muddled, but may be lucid and able to make their decision the following morning. Similarly someone may have the capacity to decide who should help with their finances, but may not be able to tell you how much money they have, what accounts they are held in, which utility companies supply their home or how much their home is worth.

The second part: does the dementia mean she is unable to make a decision? After all, Lillian *has* made a decision. She has decided she is going home. But is this a decision made with capacity? Where does a permissible 'unwise decision' end and lack of capacity start? The Mental Capacity Act requires that Lillian must be able to understand information about the decision to be made, and retain that information in her mind, and use or weigh that information as part of the decision-making process and communicate her decision.

When I go through things later with Lillian, it's clear that she doesn't understand the information she is given. She denies ever having fallen. She says I am talking nonsense. She tells me she will not fall again. I gently mention the burns on her arms, which came about when she lay against a radiator one night, and she glances at them without interest before turning to sort through the contents of her handbag once more. There is no sign that she uses or weighs information in making her decision about going home.

That district nurse, who had listened to Lillian's view that she would like to stay in her own home, was wrong to think she must have capacity. Lillian does not have capacity to decide whether to be discharged from the hospital or to live at home or move into care. She has an opinion, which is a different thing. People who have an opinion may lack capacity; people who do not have capacity may, importantly, have an opinion.

That afternoon I talk with Lillian's niece Neoma, who has driven across two counties to be here again.

'There's a groove down the road now,' Neoma says, 'from my place to Lil's and to this place.'

Neoma explains further. At the same time as refusing help Lillian has increased the rate at which she issues demands, making phone calls to the district nurses who visit to dress her injuries and to the care agency and her GP. She phones her neighbour, Helen, every few hours, and pulls the emergency cord incessantly to summon Robbie. As she has become less physically able she has become determined that others should help maintain her world exactly as she desires it. The carers have been visiting six times a day, but just as one has closed the door on her way out Lillian is on the phone to Neoma to complain that the TV listings magazine has been left open on the wrong page. Lillian's behaviour has started to fizz. In my mind I see a Catherine wheel set alight on a dark autumn evening – at first a few sparks emerge and the wheel turns slowly, then it speeds up, throwing off flashes of light, faster and faster. The audience instinctively leans backwards and hands go up to protect faces.

Neoma is a social worker herself and understands the issues. Lillian chose Neoma as her attorney in an LPA prepared years ago. 'I was quite surprised,' Neoma says.

'It was when my mum died – her sister. I think that shook her. She told me she didn't trust herself to make decisions forever. That was a rare thing for Auntie Lil to admit any vulnerability, that she could ever be wrong about something.'

Neoma knows the rules. As the attorney for health and care she can make decisions on Lillian's behalf, but that power is tempered because those who hold LPA are, like me, required to have regard to the code of practice and the Mental Capacity Act that the code supports. Neoma's decisions must be in Lillian's best interests. This means that Lillian's past and present wishes, her opinion about what's right for her, must be taken into account. And she certainly has an opinion.

The MCA demands that we seek the least restrictive option. When researching his book *Being Mortal* Atul Gawande talked with Keren Brown Wilson, one of the freedom fighters for older people in the USA, about the decisions to move people into care. Keren explained, 'We want autonomy for ourselves, and safety for those we love.' Lillian herself has scant regard for her safety.

Moving Lillian into a care home will deprive her of liberty. It is right that we should make every effort to find ways in which we can meet her needs without infringing her right to freedom. Neoma knows that.

'I really have tried for Auntie Lil,' she says.

'Everyone's done everything, I think, to keep her at home.'

Neoma sighs. 'I know she's not happy in hospital, but

the thing is, she's actually unhappy at home too. So I think she can be unhappy and unsafe at home, or unhappy but safer in a care home.'

We have a strict regard for personal liberty in the UK, and while processes can seem bureaucratic they are there to protect a vulnerable group of people. We had a problem in my hospital some years ago with the rules concerning deprivation of liberty, which were inadvertently harming a few of our patients, as there was a row about where they should be cared for while decisions were being made. I wrote to Baroness Ilora Finlay, who was chairing a review of aspects of the Mental Capacity Act, and I was invited to meet her in the House of Lords, where she gave me clear and helpful advice to solve our difficulty. But when I complained that the best interests decision-making felt to me sometimes overly ponderous, Lady Finlay fixed me with a firm gaze.

'You may think that, but I am telling you these decisions are not always made properly.' She looked at me over her glasses. 'You know what it's like in a group. You get one strong leader, and everyone else feels they have to behave like sheep.'

I was chastened. Lady Finlay was right and I knew it. I have made wrong decisions about someone's capacity before now, and have been redirected by experienced community psychiatric nurses, who listened to Enid's rambling incoherence and reinstated the antipsychotic medication that had fallen off her list somewhere between her little flat and my ward – a single transformational depot injection of a long-acting drug, due every four weeks, that had somehow dropped down the crack between primary and secondary care. I have had my view of what might be in someone's best interests challenged by strong social workers, and they have been proven correct, supporting Josiah to return to his home, even though he could not recall the name of his street or his town, and often even his own name, and could not use a phone or a lifeline alarm, but Josiah was given a full breakfast in the café opposite his flat each day and could find his way home, and the café waitress would ring his social worker if Josiah wasn't in by nine. These decisions are often more finely balanced than they appear.

In Lillian's case, however, we find unanimity. Her own social worker meets Neoma, and hears about everything that had already been tried. I ask one of the psychogeriatricians to help. He meets her and writes a short and perfect letter.

I have assessed Mrs Jason. She has dementia, and as a result she is unable to understand and weigh up information about her care. She therefore does not have capacity to make decisions about her care, even with support. There is no prospect of her regaining capacity. I believe that every effort has gone into trying less restrictive options for her care at home, and that it is now in her best interests to be cared for in a secure environment in which I believe she will benefit from attention and interaction from others.

A few days later we are waiting for a care home manager to assess Lillian.

'Nurse! Nurse!' There is a crash. Lillian is holding a spoon upright, banging it on the table. 'Nurse!'

I go to her. 'Lillian, are you all right? How can I help?'

Lillian puts the spoon down, and scowls. '*Now* whaddya want?'

*

Although the Mental Capacity Act 2005 sets out the basic legislation, it is supported by a lengthy code of practice. You can find it here:

https://www.gov.uk/government/publications/mental-capacity-act-code-of-practice

17. Attorney

I am sitting in a bright kitchen, that of Eliza, whose children go swimming with ours, and she is banging things around as she puts the kettle on and says, 'Dad –' bang, the kettle is on its connection plate – 'wants me to be his LPA thingy, attorney –' mugs are out of the cupboard and the door slams – 'and he wants my brother Sam to be the other one –' the fridge door is thrown shut, bottles clank – 'and he won't tell us what he wants, just says we'll know when the time comes –' the milk bottle bashes onto the table – 'and he knows we haven't spoken to each other for four years –' boiling water slops over the rim of the mugs – 'since the camper-van thing. It's a bloody disaster.' She pulls a chair back and sits with her elbows on the table, and holds the skin of her temples back with both hands.

It is not a good idea to try to use Lasting Power of Attorney as a tool to mend a fractured family.

Lasting Powers of Attorney (LPAs) are legal documents authorizing someone else (the attorney) to act on your behalf in England and Wales. The LPAs were created in 2005 when the Mental Capacity Act was introduced and replaced the old system of English Enduring Powers of

Attorney (EPAs). If you have an EPA, then it may still be valid but it will only deal with your finances. An EPA has no effect with regards to your welfare.

There are two types of LPA in England and Wales, one for property and financial affairs (a finance LPA), which can take effect immediately and endures if you lose capacity, and one for health and welfare (a welfare LPA, sometimes also called a health and care LPA), which only comes into effect if you lose the mental capacity to make your own welfare decisions. There is a similar system in Scotland, using slightly different nomenclature, while in Northern Ireland an EPA can confer the power to make financial decisions, but does not make provision for issues of welfare.

If you become unable to make specific decisions for yourself and if you have appointed an attorney (or more than one attorney), the attorney(s) can 'stand in your shoes'. They can make decisions for you, as if they were you, but they must ensure that they comply with the five principles of the Mental Capacity Act 2005. The attorney(s) are not allowed to make any old decision, such as one that makes their life easier but doesn't reflect your wishes. They must make decisions that are in your best interests.

Many more people prepare finance LPAs than welfare LPAs, so why should anyone appoint an attorney for their health and care? After all, without this status families and those close to a person still have a right to express their views about what that person would have wanted, and those views must be heard and taken into account, and many medical decisions are clear cut, and a medical team will be able to explain to those people what is the right thing to do. But many decisions are not so clear and the outcome turns on a person's values, which may be held in their heart and shared with only a few very close people. So for those possible future decisions, which may indeed be finely balanced, many prefer that the final arbiter will be someone they trust, whom they have appointed themselves. People choose to do this at different stages in their lives. A few with a lively distrust of the medical profession set up an LPA while they are in youthful good health. Others appoint an LPA for health and care when some shadow falls across their lives, a diagnosis like a stroke or dementia, that might presage vulnerability.

Although giving someone LPA for health and care can make things go more smoothly when you can't make your own decisions, there's still plenty of scope for argument about what your best interests might actually be. If, like Eliza's father, you must appoint warring parties, at least give them a working plan upon which to base their peace talks, because attorneys who have not agreed with one another about anything for several years are likely to find it hard to come to an agreement about you. If having a conversation with your attorneys about your wishes is impossible – too sensitive, too inflammatory – you can set out your views in a Letter of Wishes, and you can tell your attorneys where they can find that letter should the need arise for them to act together on your behalf. That is a kind thing to do, to keep the petrol away from the bonfire that you may have inadvertently built, but it is even kinder to go through that letter with your attorneys face to face.

The next problem is that LPA can be a clumsy tool in an emergency. It may happen that an emergency arises, and there is dispute about quick decisions that need to be taken, right now, and a brother in Northampton phones to say he is one attorney and a sister in Leeds says, 'No, he isn't. I didn't know anything about that.' A medical team is left in an awkward position because we can check with the Office of the Public Guardian whether an LPA is registered and they 'will respond within five working days'. Five working days! For emergency care you need an emergency healthcare plan or a TEP, which can stand alongside the details you've put into your welfare LPA. You can give a copy of your welfare LPA to your GP so that it sits within your medical records, but a complete copy of the welfare LPA, even in the medical records, is often not fully accessible in an emergency – a locally accepted TEP or emergency healthcare plan is a safer bet. If you update the LPA, it is vital that you remember to update the version held by your GP.

A third problem arises when your attorneys are unaware of your wishes.

A woman was standing at the foot of a bed when my youngest trainee Saida and I arrived on the acute medical unit, and I was already taking a phone call from a worried GP about someone quite different, a patient at home, so I was listening to that GP while I watched the woman, who was in distress. She put her handbag on the bed and picked it up, then put it back down and put her hands together, her index fingers on her lips, and took a deep breath and brought her hands apart, then she breathed out and her hands went back together, and she knocked her fingers on her lips three times. It was clear that a decision, or its consequences, was troubling her, and her turmoil was very sad to see.

A few minutes later we met Ivan, who was very sick – sick enough to die. He was peacefully unconscious, oblivious to the drip in his arm and the antibiotics running through it, and we met Abigail, who wept as she explained that she was welfare LPA for Ivan, her step-father, and she had discovered only that morning when the nursing home had rung to say he was ill, that he had made a plan with his GP, which specified that he did not want to go to hospital should he become unwell.

Abigail went on, coiling a paper tissue in her hands. 'I know he meant what he said with the GP. I'm sure that *was* what he said then, but it's my duty to protect him because now he can't speak for himself and he trusted me . . . he *trusted* me to be his attorney, and I rang a solicitor after the home called me and they said I could override his plan if I thought it was right to do that, so I did. I made them call an ambulance and now he's here and I don't know if I have done right.'

And all of that situation took a lot of untangling, and a conversation with Abigail about what had been happening in Ivan's life and what was important to him, and whether the plan he had made was indeed the right plan. We tried to establish whether it was a decision about not coming to hospital that Ivan had made with capacity, which should have been respected, even though Abigail felt it was a wrong decision; or whether Ivan had perhaps not had capacity when he talked with his GP. So there was a phone call to that doctor to check what he and Ivan had discussed, and why Ivan felt the way he did, then more reassurance to Abigail that she had done what she felt was best at the time, as she had been placed in an almost impossible position.

The rules concerning the interaction between a welfare LPA and plans made with medical teams, such as an emergency healthcare plan, a TEP or an Advance Decision to Refuse Treatment (ADRT) are complicated. If you make a legally valid ADRT, and then appoint someone as your welfare power of attorney, then your welfare attorney is technically allowed to override your ADRT. If, on the other hand, you appoint a welfare attorney and *then* make an ADRT, your welfare attorney must abide by the subsequent ADRT that sets out your decision to refuse treatment. Other medical plans, things like resus decisions and emergency health plans, aren't specifically covered by the Mental Capacity Act; they are plans that reflect your wishes and should be considered when deciding what is in your best interests. It's hard for your welfare attorney to act in your best interests if they don't know what your wishes are. It may well be that Ivan had wanted to protect Abigail from the knowledge that he did not want active treatment, or maybe he feared that she would try to talk him out of his plans, or maybe he did not really think through his emergency plan and its ramifications for Abigail. I do not know, but in the end it would have been better if Abigail had known about his wishes and in particular his plans for care in an emergency. Abigail could then have had time to come to terms with what Ivan desired for his own future treatment.

Your attorneys need to be aware of your wishes particularly if you specify that you want them to be able to make decisions about emergency care and especially about life-prolonging treatment, which would include, for example, decisions about being fed by tube or being taken to hospital in case of life-threatening illness. Your attorneys must know where to find your LPA document and they need to be aware of its contents, and of the wishes you've included in any Letter of Wishes, TEP form, ADRT or associated advance care plan.

The final complication concerning health and welfare powers of attorney is perhaps more readily solved by being alert to the possibility that care may need paying for, and making it easier for your welfare attorney to do that. In the case of Neoma, trying to keep up with her aunt Lil's rapidly escalating needs for care, it made all the difference that Lil had granted her an LPA for finances as well as an LPA for health and welfare. An LPA for finance can be used as soon as it is registered with the Office of the Public Guardian, provided the donor agrees to this (LPAs for welfare cannot be activated until the donor loses their capacity to make the relevant decisions). Thus, as a financial attorney Neoma was noted at the bank as Lil's attorney and was therefore able to do her online shopping and pay her utility bills. Neoma could also issue payments to Lil's multitude of carers, and, later on, she was able to authorize the sale of her flat so that her care home bills could be met. Without the financial LPA Neoma's life, which was complicated in any case, would have become a terrible tightening net of legal fees and bureaucracy.

For several years now I have driven past a house in a nearby village that stands empty, and I know that Joanie, who once lived there, now whiles away her days in a bright care home, while her financial arrangements are picked over by the team of the Office of the Public Guardian and the bills to her sister-in-law mount up, as that sister-in-law has kindly stepped forward to be a deputy for Joanie, and the weeds straggle by the front door that was Joanie's.

A deputy is similar to an attorney but is appointed by the Court of Protection when someone lacks capacity to make their own decisions but has not, for whatever reason, nominated a person through LPA to deal with their affairs. Joanie's sister-in-law has had to instruct a solicitor and pay their fees and court fees, which stack up rapidly, so that she can be legally approved by the court as the right person to manage Joanie's affairs now that she cannot make decisions for herself. And although they will, for a fee, make Joanie's sister-in-law a deputy for her financial affairs, the Court of Protection is reluctant to appoint welfare deputies, falling back instead on 'best interests' principles for decisions about Joanie's health and care, so her sister-in-law can only contribute a view to those discussions rather than having the right to make decisions as if she was in Joanie's shoes.

Your LPA for finances and your LPA for health and welfare do not need to be the same person, but they do need to be able to work together. Granting someone power of attorney for welfare without a parallel arrangement for finances is generally a mistake; it may land responsibilities upon that attorney without giving them the tools necessary to act upon those responsibilities.

I talk to Sally, who is a solicitor with an intricate understanding of powers of attorney, deputyships, trusts and the execution of wills, and who deals with the administration of people's estates (often called probate – obtaining a Grant of Probate is the legal process of 'proving' a will). She is a member of two associations that offer further training and qualifications to solicitors working in this area. Sally sighs. I can hear her concern as we speak on the phone. Sally explains, 'I say sorting out LPA, especially for finances, is like getting your hair cut. You can do it yourself, and it will be a hair cut and it won't be perfect, but it will hopefully be better than nothing. You may make a mess of it and have to get the mess you created sorted out professionally. Or you can decide to get professional help in the first place. There is no doubt that instructing a qualified expert solicitor will be more expensive than doing it yourself, but it may save money in the long run. Regardless of whether your affairs are simple or complicated, it's easy to get it wrong, and that can get expensive quickly. It's a very personal decision but one that needs proper consideration.'

Sally points out some of the easy mistakes people can make. One is the decision whether to appoint attorneys to make decisions 'jointly or severally' or 'jointly'. Often people think that 'jointly' sounds like a good idea, because then their attorneys have to agree before making the decisions on their behalf. However, Sally goes on to say, 'a joint decision made without proper advice can be a disaster, because if one of your joint attorneys dies, or goes bankrupt if they're a financial attorney, the whole joint appointment is a write-off and the other joint attorney(s) can't act for you. This may mean that in practical terms you now have no attorney appointed. For this reason a "joint and several" appointment can be considered safer.' Whichever type of LPA you create it is wise and kind to give your attorneys guidance about your wishes. They may have to make important decisions on your behalf. It may be difficult to discuss these sensitive sad possibilities, but it is vital for the attorney to understand what your wishes are if they need to act as if they were you.

Conversely if you are asked to act as an attorney, it is reasonable to have a careful conversation about their wishes with the person who has asked you to make decisions on their behalf so that you may feel confident that you are indeed 'standing in their shoes' when the time comes.

The clue is in the name. Creation of an LPA confers power, the power to make important decisions on behalf of another person. With power comes responsibility. It is responsible to be bold and start the conversation, in both directions, and to write this conversation down if you are able, so that you are confident that your attorney can follow your wishes. In turn, if you are that attorney, you will have the comfort of knowing that the decisions you make are those that would have been wanted.

*

You can find the information to appoint an LPA here: https://www.gov.uk/government/publications/make-a-lasting-power-of-attorney

The societies that offer extra training and qualifications for UK solicitors dealing with LPA are Solicitors for the Elderly (SFE, a group of qualified solicitors who are experts in dealing with older adults) and STEP (Society of Trust and Estate Practitioners, again qualified solicitors who are experts on tax, trusts, probate and accounts). Both SFE and STEP have pages on their websites to enable you to find a qualified solicitor in your area.

https://sfe.legal
https://www.step.org

Any solicitor you consult should be registered with the Law Society. You can find one here:

https://solicitors.lawsociety.org.uk/

18. Not Lost

It's a Saturday afternoon and the children are bundled in their coats against a biting March wind as they dangle upside down from our tatty climbing frame. I'm not on call, but the phone rings, and it is Leon, ringing from the community hospital. He is soft-spoken and thoughtful, deferential.

'I am sorry to disturb you, doctor, but we have lost a patient.'

My heart turns over. The community hospital is newly reopened after some years of dereliction, and I'm aware that the security system for the doors hasn't yet been installed.

'Who is it?' I ask.

'Mr Kiston. Room Four.'

Oh, poor man. He was so frail when I last saw him, but comfortable, asleep much of the day. What can have happened? I picture him walking unsteadily through the little car park on to the road – there might be traffic. Oh God, there's a ditch, deep. Mud, water. And it's so cold . . .

'Where have you looked? Have you called the police?'

There's a pause. 'No, doctor. We have lost him. He is dead. It was peaceful.'

I watch the children. My son is on one end of a moulded plastic see-saw, trying to bounce his sisters into the air. There are squeals. I breathe. Mr Kiston, Clifford, not lost but dead.

Dr Kathryn Mannix has a kind and sensible voice, and what she says is kind and sensible. She is a palliative care consultant and has spent her working life with those who are dying. Her book, *With the End in Mind*, tells compassionate stories of 'ordinary people dying', drawn from a deep well of experience. Kathryn's on a mission to help people approach death without being afraid. In a BBC video she describes a normal death, and I cannot do better than her words.

'Dying, like giving birth, is just a process. With time people become more tired, more weary. As time goes by people sleep more, and they're awake less. At some point a family or carer might go to give them a medicine, or they have a visitor. But this time, when we go to wake the person who is dying, they are more than asleep, they are unconscious and can't be woken.'

Kathryn explains why this is important, speaking slowly and clearly. There are pauses between her sentences. She says, 'And that's when we realize that a change has taken place. It's tiny but it's really significant, because instead of being just asleep, the person has temporarily become unconscious. We can't wake them up.'

She explains what this experience, this unconsciousness close to death, is like for her patients.

'And yet when they waken later on they say they have had a good sleep. So we know that this coma when someone is dying is not frightening, that lapsing into unconsciousness just isn't noticed by us when it happens. As time goes by the person who is dying is awake less and asleep more, until eventually they're just unconscious all the time.'

Kathryn goes on to describe some of the things that frighten people who are present when they don't know about normal dying. She says, 'The person who is dying will be so relaxed that they won't bother to clear their throat, so maybe they'll be breathing in and out through little bits of saliva at the back of their throat and it makes a rattly noise. People talk about the death rattle as though it's something terrible, but actually it tells me that my patient is so deeply relaxed, so deeply unconscious, that they're not even feeling that tickle of saliva as the air bubbles through it in and out of their lungs.'

At the very end of somebody's life there will be a period of shallow breathing, then sometimes there is an out breath, and no in breath for what seems like an age. Have they died? Suddenly there may be another deep breath, and the dying person breathes again, perhaps a few big breaths, then slower and shallower breaths for a while, and then stops breathing once more. Sometimes that cycle – of shallow breath, no breath, big breath – can go on for a long time, hours or even days.

Kathryn explains, 'And then there is one out breath that just isn't followed by another in breath. Sometimes it's so gentle that families don't even notice that it's happened.'

Her explanation is kind. And it is true. She says, 'Normal human dying is just a really gentle process, one that we can recognize, something we can prepare for, something we can manage.'

This is not to say that death is uncomplicated, or that a final illness doesn't come with symptoms like pain, nausea or breathlessness. But these are symptoms of illness, not of dying itself. These symptoms of illness require attention, expertise, palliation. The process of death, however . . . for that we need a conversation.

'Janet, you are not going to die.' Not like this, not right now. Janet needs to know that her death is not going to happen this way.

She is clinging on to the rails on each side of her bed. The side room on the acute medical unit is filled with noise: the NIV apparatus strapped to Janet's face is hissing furiously and two women – one in a coat, the other in a dressing gown, in their forties or fifties maybe – are crying in one another's arms. A son – son-in-law? – is on his phone to someone else, arguing about whether they should come in. The monitor reads Janet's dismal oxygen levels from her finger and beeps incessantly. I turn off the sound – the numbers are clear enough.

I usher the son out of the room and smile at the daughters and give them a thumbs up. Surprised, they stop their noisy crying and turn to look at their mum.

Janet's eyes are popping with fear and effort. Her face is red with broken veins. Her hair is a rigid frizz. The room smells sweaty, full of dismay.

'Janet, can you hear me?' I introduce myself. 'I know this is very scary, but it is going to be all right.'

Janet's eyes bulge as she shakes her head. Not all right. Her shoulders are rounded, plumped by years of high-dose steroids, and her arms are thin. Her fists twist outwards to grip the bed rails, and her skin is white around each thumbnail. Nando is with me, and I say, 'Nando, there should be some opiate on her drug chart, please can you get it? And can you ask someone who knows about NIV to pop in?'

NIV, non-invasive ventilation – oxygen run at high pressure through a tight-fitting mask – was introduced after my registrar years, and I've never really got the hang of it, but I know it shouldn't be making this much racket.

'Janet, I'm just going to –' I prise her hand from the rail, lowering it so I can perch on the bed – 'do this.'

I hold her right hand in my right hand, as if we are about to arm-wrestle, and say, 'You are doing so well,' and I look into her eyes, which are very, very frightened, and the tears are wet on her face above the tight mask.

'Janet, I can see that you think you are going to die,' and she looks at me and nods, and I hear a squeak from one of the daughters, so I turn to them, and ask, 'Is that how you're feeling too?' They nod, and one clasps the hand of her sister, and I ask if they could move the chairs a little so they can sit by their mum's head, where I can see them too, while I'm talking to her.

'Janet, I know you have been very ill for a long time, and your lungs are terrible, and I know you know that, and you've talked with Dr Telford about it.'

Janet nods and breathes even faster.

'So you and I both know that your lungs aren't going to keep going for ever.' I squeeze her hand. 'And I can see you are very sick this time, and I think you might be right that this time you might be going to die.'

Janet's mouth opens for a few panted breaths, then closes as she sniffs in, out, in, out through her nose again. Her daughters shuffle closer to one another.

'But you are not going to die like this, all scared.'

Janet turns her head and closes her eyes. She's exhausted, but her eyes fly open again and she shifts her body with an effort to try to get more air.

'Janet, I want to tell you about something, because I think it will make you feel better. I can see that you're thinking each breath you take now is going to be your last breath –' she stares at me and widens her eyes as she nods in agreement – 'and that's a horrible feeling, but it's not going to be like that.'

She keeps her gaze on me and the machine hisses. One lock of her frizzy hair is stuck down on to her forehead, and I smooth it away with my thumb.

'Janet. And Janet's girls. We're going to fix this mask so it's not so noisy, and we're going to give you a tiny dose of morphine, which is not enough to knock you out, just enough to take the edge off this scary breathing. OK?'

There are more nods.

'And then you'll feel a bit better. Janet, you're not going to die gasping. Do you mind if I tell you what's going to happen when the time comes for you to die?'

And she nods again and squeezes my hand, and I bow my head a little to her daughters, to check with them, and they hold each other, and I explain that in the end, maybe this time, maybe another time, when she's ready, when she and her team have decided that treatment's not helping, we'll take off that tight mask, and stop checking her oxygen levels over and over, because none of us will worry what her oxygen level is and we'll help her breathing with an ordinary mask, or even with just a fan, and I explain that she will be able to relax, and to sleep, and that her sleep will be peaceful, and that she might wake up again, then sleep some more, and at some point in one of those deep sleeps, when she is not conscious, she will breathe out, very gently, and then she will not breathe in again.

And at some point in that conversation Sean has arrived, who is one of the critical care outreach nurses, and I love that team, for he swiftly fits the NIV mask more snugly round Janet's chin and adjusts the pressures on the machine, and the racket stops and is replaced by a quieter whooshing.

Then Nando comes in with a very small dose of

morphine in a syringe, and I say, 'I think maybe just half of that now, Nando.' Because Janet's breathing has slowed down, and the oxygen levels on her monitor are creeping up and Janet's death isn't going to happen right now, but when it does, and after perhaps several more conversations like this one, she and her family will be ready for it and will manage.

There is another thing about death, which I think is easily overlooked, because it is one of the great differences between very old people and the younger people who look after them, and that is faith. For faith is a rock-solid certainty for many of my patients, and the meaning of faith, its rituals and hymns or chants or prayers, are woven into them, and younger people may have that to some degree, but often a great deal less than their parents or grandparents, or do not have faith at all, or even find faith positively objectionable, and it's easy to forget that faith for many isn't just a Sunday thing or a visit to a synagogue or a mosque on special occasions, but is absolutely the warp and weft of life. And, my goodness, death is one of the moments in life when faith does its stuff, and belief transcends all physical concerns and lifts someone so gently and tenderly out of this world and into eternity. It's there on our end-of-life care form, which asks 'Have the patient's spiritual needs been met?' And I know, I *know*, it is glossed over for I have glossed over it myself. Sometimes I have asked a family 'Would your father or mother like to see a chaplain?' and been given a funny look, which has knocked me back, and I have felt embarrassed and worried that I might have offended that family, and perhaps the next time I would not ask, and would pretend to myself that perhaps one of the nurses should ask that question not me.

Edward lay on my ward, dying with cancer quietly and slowly for a week or so, and he was very alone in the world and mumbled from time to time when he wakened and looked anxiously past our shoulders when we tried to discern what it was that troubled him, and his distress became more and more apparent, and more and more impossible to fathom, until one day his cleaner visited, bringing Edward his post, which included a card from his church, and I rang the hospital chaplaincy and one of the chaplains came up to the ward and said prayers with Edward and gave him communion, after which Edward slept, and slept some more, and died, and that is a true story.

Edward is not the only person for whom faith, in the end, was the single most important thing. He is one of many, and my grandmother breathed her life slowly away over several days. Even after her daughters were assembled she breathed some more, until late one day my grandfather recited to her the liturgy of the Anglican Evening Prayer, which he knew by heart and which includes the Nunc Dimittis, 'Lord, now lettest thou thy servant depart in peace . . . for mine eyes have seen thy salvation.' That was when my grandmother breathed out and did not need to take another breath.

I no longer gloss over that question of spiritual needs. I would rather slightly offend someone who is not bothered about faith than miss the moment for someone to whom faith is all-important. Most often a family know exactly where someone's beliefs lie, but occasionally they may need a prompt to consider that, although they themselves may feel that the divine is not present in their lives, and their parent or grandparent may even no longer attend a place of worship, yet faith may be present still, and needs to be respected and given space to do its beautiful, peaceful and loving thing, whether or not we bystanders choose to believe.

Here is another thing about death. Sometimes we think we recognize it, but we are wrong. One morning we are jammed into the treatment room – a staff nurse, OT, physio, social worker, discharge liaison worker, two junior doctors, me. Our ward sister Linda keeps an eye on us as we run through the list of patients on a whiteboard, the jobs for the day – who is sick, who is new, what needs doing to help someone get home – and from time to time another nurse squeezes in, sorry, sorry, to get something from a drug cupboard. We reach Pat, who is in a side room, and Linda says, 'That family's not happy.' I put my head on one side to hear why, and Linda says, 'She looked as if she was going again last night so we called them in, and she's brighter this morning.'

And I feel sorry for Pat's family, and sorry for the nurses, because this is the second time the family has been called to her bedside to say goodbye and we've been wrong. She is at the end of her illness with dementia and has not walked for nearly a year, nor spoken, and at her best now Pat is asleep much of the day, waking to take a mouthful of soup, a teaspoon of porridge. How can that be enough to sustain her? She does not move really, or make a sound, but she wrinkles her round face into an appreciative expression, then drifts off to sleep again, and the pneumonia has surged, making her nose icy to touch, lips blue, breath so shallow it's hardly there; then the infection has ebbed away, despite no treatment, as her small doughty body chugs along, churning out white cells that must be made of thin air. We'd made plans for her to get back to her nursing home, to die there, 'where the duvet matches the curtains', and the ambulance transport was booked for today, but last night she looked to be at the end, her breathing cycling, great pauses of long minutes where there was no breath at all, and we don't – putting it frankly – we don't want her to die in the ambulance, so we're all waiting, not just Pat's family. And now, this morning, she's had three, four sips of sugary tea, and has given the care assistant a gummy grin and she is asleep again, her soft cheeks pale but pink, and I don't know. I honestly don't know. Usually we see death approaching and recognize him, but sometimes he is a sheep in wolf's clothing and comes trotting towards us then turns away. Sometimes a family member like Pat's son may be far away, working – he has a big job – and he wonders whether to come, and I have to make a judgement, and say, if there are things unsaid, reasons that you need to be at your mother's side at the end, then it is better perhaps that you come now, for I would rather you were here, watching her get better, than far away and hearing she has died. And sometimes we will have a rueful smile together when I've got it wrong (I find myself apologizing that someone has not died), and that son might joke gently that he reckons it's the littlest old ladies that are most difficult to call, and he might well be right.

In someone who has cancer the signs that death is imminent include profound weakness, a small appetite, sleepiness – but these are features of everyday life in someone who is very frail. Being muddled, becoming quiet, not responding to things people are saying or to music or a familiar face – those might be new signs in someone who until recently was vibrant, and suggest that death is approaching. But in those who are most frail, especially people who have dementia as well, that state of withdrawal from the world may last a long time. Perhaps it is those who are frailest, those who have been hovering between earth and sky for some time, who catch us out and hover a little longer.

'Can he hear me?' asks Wendy, and I have to say I do not know. As Kathryn Mannix observes, often a person who is dying will awaken transiently from a period of deep sleep that may have been unconsciousness and has no recollection of anything, no dream, no troubling thought, no music or voices. Yet sometimes a person may be just exhausted, resting, eyes closed, while they are also dying, and of course they can hear. So I smile when I am about to enter a room and I hear low voices talking about lives together, silly happy things, and a meal that went wrong, or a journey, and the time someone fell out of a tree.

There are some practical questions that come up. Please may I donate my body or parts of my body, or am I too old? To which the answers are, no, you are not too old, and, yes, you may donate at any age, and I talk to the bequest office at one medical school, through which people may donate their bodies for medical students and surgeons that they may learn, and the administrator tells me that her oldest donor was 105, and another office's record holder was 103. Plans for this process need to be made in advance, and if there is a family they must of course be involved. It is not age that precludes donation, but many conditions do, such as a history of TB (because the tubercle bacillus can lie dormant for decades).

UK organ donation is in the process of becoming 'opt out', but families will still have the last say on all donation, so it's wise to ensure that our families know our wishes. The organ donation team also helps with gifts of smaller parts of ourselves, and there are no age restrictions for donations of bone, skin or eyes. The team need to be notified quickly after a death that someone who wishes to be a donor has died, and they can be rung by anyone, hospital staff, family or friends. But even when someone hopes to have donated all or some part of themselves things can go awry at the end, which may be a disappointment, and the Parkinson's UK Brain Bank team (which is one of many potential recipients of such donations) puts it kindly when they explain that 'the circumstances that may prevent collection do not reduce the value of the intended donation, the spirit in which the gift was made, or the efforts made by the donor's next of kin to fulfil the donor's wishes.'

After a death, responsibility for care of what was a person and is now a body, shifts from the Department of Health to the Ministry of Justice, and the interface between the two organizations can be a hard place for those who are bereaved. My patient James was shaken after his wife of sixty-two years died, and at a time when he did not need more shaking, by a telephone call from the coroner's office quizzing him on the manner of her death. For the coroner has an interest in deaths that might be termed unnatural, and your and my idea of what might be unnatural isn't quite the same as that of the Ministry of Justice. James's wife Em had stumbled while shopping and had fallen, scraping her leg on a kerb. It had bled a bit, but they had cleaned it up together and put a dressing on it, and a week or so later she'd caught her hand lifting a pan from an awkward cupboard, and she had a bit of a scab there too, and she already had dodgy kidneys that didn't bother her too much and she was a bit slowed up by her heart and she had a chronic grumbling problem with her bone marrow with imperfect quality control, so the red cells sent out by her marrow were misshapen and in short supply, and her white cells, which should combat infection, didn't work perfectly either. Em had woken after a nap one afternoon shivering and grey, and James had called an ambulance right then, which arrived promptly and took Em to hospital, where antibiotics were shot into her vein even as the team were listening to her story. Despite this her heart, lungs, kidneys, brain and eventually life itself fell like dominoes to an overwhelming infection. It wasn't clear where the infection had come from – it might have been pneumonia or a urine infection, but it might have been from one of those scrapes on her leg or her hand, which were caused by trauma. A death of someone whose body is already frail from a sudden severe infection could not be a more natural death. But any death that is *due to (that is, more than minimally, negligibly or trivially), caused, or contributed to by . . . violence, trauma or physical injury*, including *violence, trauma or physical injury sustained in an accident such as a fall*, is a death that must be notified to the coroner, and Em's death was eventually declared 'accidental' rather than 'natural', which was upsetting for James, as somehow there seemed to be an implication that he might have prevented Em's stumble or lifted that pan out himself, because an accident always sounds like something that could have been averted.

There is tension between three threads. There is the need for accuracy of death certificates and this pulls against the uncertainty that features more often in medicine than we'd like. And perhaps tugging in a slightly different direction are the concerns of a widower, son or friend, who is left behind and is trying to make sense of what happened. Different hospitals have different systems for who decides what to put on a certificate, and soon we shall have medical examiners who will adjudicate, but even then there'll be room for interpretation of the facts and another person might have ascribed Em's death to some other source of infection and that would have been a natural death, and wouldn't need to trouble the coroner at all. And similarly it's not always clear what someone has actually died of, when that person is very old and very frail, and some doctors will allow 'frailty of old age' on a certificate, and others will not, insisting that we make a best guess, put ischaemic heart disease or a heart attack, even when we know that someone's end may have been both more complicated, and simpler, than that.

My stepfather died while I've been writing this book, and that trip to Costa Rica was his last big trip abroad, although he returned every June to Caen in Normandy, and to the broad empty beach and the land in between that was shelled by the gun he commanded at nineteen years old in 1944, when the sky was dark with planes and the beach was deep in horror, and torpedoes sped, visible in the water, past his ship to sink the Norwegian vessel beside his own. In his desk after he'd died was an A4 notebook on which he had written *What Happens Next* neatly, and inside was the name of his solicitor and where to find his will. And his bank details: account numbers for each utility company; the location of the mains stopcock in the bungalow should a pipe burst; the charities he supported, which might benefit from any donations. His choice of funeral director; the name of the vicar and the church – though Mum knew that, but had she been unable to speak he had it covered. There was the contact number for the chairman of the association of those who had served in his very first ship, the chairman who arranges annual gatherings of shipmates (though my stepfather's are all gone now and it's a society of younger men, and women these days, who had been welcoming him still). And later on in his book were hymns, readings and prayers, snipped out from the funeral service sheets of friends and glued with Pritt Stick to the pages.

To envisage the disarray that his death would create and to put in place soft buffers against which our grief could bump, that was a kind thing to do. Some of the components of his funeral service were included too, I think as an offering to his friends, because the younger people attending may have been there to mourn a very old man, but even at ninety-four there were, as he knew there may be, some present who were mourning the friend of their youth. Even when someone is very old, loss remains loss.

*

You can watch Dr Mannix talk about the process of death here:
  https://www.bbc.com/ideas/videos/dying-is-not-as-bad-as-you-think/po62moxt

You can find out about donating your body to a medical school via the Human Tissue Authority here. Be warned, this needs to be set up in advance of a death.
  https://www.hta.gov.uk/medical-schools

The organ donor team and their phone number can be found at
  https://www.organdonation.nhs.uk/register-to-donate/

19. Lap of Honour

'Oh, tell that man I love him,' says Harriet. 'I haven't even met him, and I love him already.'

Harriet is a psychogeriatrician, and I have been talking to her about George Coxon, with whom I have a meeting later that day at the care home he owns. George's home specializes in the care of those who have dementia, and his team ticks all the boxes to keep their residents safe. Rated 'outstanding' at its most recent inspection, in George's home risks are assessed and medicines well managed. Staff are carefully recruited and trained, and in the words of the inspection report, everyone knows 'their responsibilities to safeguard vulnerable people'.

But George has had enough of safeguarding. His team does it perfectly, but it's not enough. George is into fun-guarding. That afternoon I arrive at the home. The exterior paint is peeling and there are weeds in the gravel of the car park, which is shared with some bins. The bell is answered by 'another George', who introduces himself and ushers me in. I meet Jan, who makes me a cup of tea. The corridors are narrow and there is stuff everywhere. Books, toys, trophies. Paintings. Dice. Tennis balls. Maracas. Photos with titles: Ivy winning the cup-stacking contest; David, the conker champion. A photo of a child, watched by a very old woman as she concentrates on a shove-ha'penny board, on which instead of coins there are jelly babies. A picture of a ballerina, underneath which a label asks: *This painting is by Edgar Degas – was he German, French or Dutch?* There is a small garden, two chickens in a run, a rabbit hutch. There are homemade posters announcing outings, anniversaries.

One of the posters is a tribute to Tom Kitwood, a social scientist and professor of psychogerontology, pioneer of a 'person-centred' approach to people living with dementia. Kitwood encouraged carers to develop their intuitive, emotional responses, in order that they would find it natural to treat others in a way they themselves would like to be treated. By coincidence, Tom Kitwood almost shares his name with another hero in the field of gerontology, Tom Kirkwood. I love Professor Kirkwood's work too. It includes a famous study of older residents of Newcastle, which discovered, among a spectacular array of data, that 78% of eighty-five-year-olds rated their health as good, very good or excellent compared to others of the same age. This was, as Prof. Kirkwood reported, 'a delightful statistical impossibility that overturns the general view that life in advanced old age is made miserable by poor health.'

On another wall of George Coxon's home a display announces that it is *Time to think about bathing costumes. Did you have one like this or this?* The swimming outfits of the 1950s are great – there is boning and structure, and there are winsome flowery bathing caps. There is also a photo, taken this summer, of two people being whooshed in fat-tyred wheelchairs, by two young people in wet-suits into a foamy sea. The wheelchair pair are wearing ordinary clothes, but their bare feet stick out, held above the cold waves using strength undreamed of. Grey hair blows backwards. Everyone in the picture is making a noise, you can tell – an ooh or an ahh, a laugh or a shout. There is exhilaration.

I heard a story once about a young woman. It was the first time that she and her husband would have all the family over for Christmas Day and she was determined to do it properly, so she set to with a will, ordering a tur-key and making a pudding into which she pressed coins that she had scrubbed, and she bought a great ham and requested that her husband saw the bone off it before she baked it. Then there was a to-do, finding a suitable implement, and her husband started sawing at the bone and it was more difficult than it looked, and there was some swearing and he straightened up and said, 'Why am I doing this?' To which she replied, 'Mum always sawed the bone off; it's how you do the ham.'

And he said, 'No, let's ask your mum.'

So they rang her mum, who told them, 'You always saw the bone off the ham. *My* mother sawed the bone off the ham.'

And the young woman and her husband were going to visit Granny anyway, who was great-grandmother to their little children, and the little children ran around the nursing home while their parents sat with that very old lady and asked her, 'Why do we have to saw the bone off the ham?'

The very old lady narrowed her eyes and thought back and smiled. She said, 'Ah, you see, when I was a young woman and was first married we had a very small oven.'

'Why am I doing this?' is an excellent question. I was taught many years ago to ask it of myself over and over – a sage physician advised putting the emphasis on each word separately: 'Why *am* I doing this?'; 'Why am *I* doing this?' Challenge the status quo, he told us. Question the guideline. Think about whether this treatment – this standard procedure, this reflexive response – is right for my patient – the individual, the person.

Collectively we are beginning to ask ourselves this question about long lives, challenging ourselves to approach old age differently with creativity and ingenuity. *Why are we doing this?* we wonder, when we recognize the ageism that can shut people away from work and communities, from fun, adventure and excitement.

How can we do things differently? we ask as we realize that longevity should be a windfall, a bonus, something to treasure and enjoy.

I've been shopping and have picked up some things for Mum (sliced ham, tinned peaches, multivitamins) alongside my list (halloumi, lentils, cumin seeds). At the

checkout Alan offers to help me pack. He is neat in a
suit, smiling; there's an enamel forget-me-not flower on
his lapel. We talk about his job. Alan explains, 'I retired,
you see, from the cheese processing, and I couldn't be
retired, so I got this job, customer service. I love it.'

I admire his lapel badge, the symbol of the Alzheimer's Society. Alan tells me, 'I got it when I did the
dementia training. Jenny was in charge of that.'

He nods his head to indicate Jenny, working at the
next counter. Her big rings glint as her competent hands
flash items past the scanner. Alan continues, 'I've learned
a lot. You see it all. There's a man comes in three times
each day, paper and a bun first thing, sandwich at lunchtime, then later on he's back for something for tea, and
I told my wife and she says, "Don't you see, he's not
shopping. He's visiting the shop, visiting you lot working there." So I talked to him and it turns out his wife
has dementia. She won't come out, but he needs to get
out and see people and we talk every day now about
what he's getting for her, and he might get her to come
to the memory café in the high street one day.'

In turn I tell Alan about a man I met from another
town, who had frontotemporal dementia that had stolen
away all his words, except for 'well done, well done', and
that man used to shop with his wife, but she had died
and after that he still shopped each day on his own,
wandering into the supermarket and selecting his
favourites – an egg salad sandwich, a chocolate rice
pudding – before wandering out without paying. And I

explain to Alan how the staff there knew him and chatted to him and kept a tactful tally of his purchases, and his daughter visited every Saturday from the city and settled the bill. Alan laughs, and says he's going to tell Jenny about that.

We are finding our way towards a perception of longevity as an opportunity. Alan himself is past statutory retirement age, but he has joined the growing band of people who have chosen to work, and has been given the opportunity to do so. He has found an 'encore career' that harnesses his time and his talent (for Alan is talented – his talent is his interest in others, his concern for their well-being). Employers are opening their eyes to the accumulated knowledge that older workers can bring. At the same time there's the start of a growing understanding in our society's approach to the very oldest, the most frail.

After my meeting with George Coxon (he arrived a little late, breathless, welcoming, hands held up in apology), I look through the notes I've scribbled. Words jump from the pages. *Curiosity. Motivation. Empathy. Interaction. Respect. Thrill. Laughter. Excitement. Danger.* George isn't reckless. He speaks of being 'risk aware rather than risk averse', and he knows that his approach needs to encourage and include rather than insist. As one of his residents admonished him, 'I'm eighty-seven, and I don't need to be shaking a tambourine all day.' There is time for rest in the afternoon, and space to step away from the thrum.

I describe George's home later to my mother and she frowns.

'I'm not sure I'd like that,' she says.

'What would you prefer?' I ask her.

'I'd like a quiet place, where I can finish a book in peace,' says Mum, and I know she's right, for despite her adventuresome past she is tired and values contemplation and the shine of raindrops on an alchemilla leaf. She has already chosen the home she would prefer should she need one, its atmosphere monastic.

'And nice carers,' Mum adds, and I read out to her what George has told me of his staff. I've pressed him to explain what he means by the 'investment in staff development', which was praised in the home's inspection report, and he has described the in-house training programme, with a bonus shared out at Christmas between those who've attended all the sessions; the visits of staff to and from other homes locally; the process of 'appreciative enquiry' that allows carers to smile about their work, and to think about ways they feel they could do better.

I read to Mum George's determination that the staff of his home should be 'proud, kind, keen, interested, cheerful, caring'. He explains how time is made for talking – real talking – between staff and residents. He describes 'discovery conversations'. Every one of the home's employees is working towards a further qualification. They learn from experts who give their time, and from one another, and they learn, day by day, from the people for whom they care. There is a willingness to learn, a determination that things can be done differently.

George has given me a list of some of those by whom he is inspired. Many of the names are familiar to me: these are people working in countless places – communities, care homes, social work offices, general practice, universities, charities, hospitals – to change the picture.

There is an article in the paper about a school where a sixth-former invited a lonely widowed man to lunch with him in the canteen, and the old man now has lunch there every week. It's a heart-warming story, but why is it a story? We can make this happen in every school, every week, and for more than one lonely person at a time. We do not need to separate those who are very old from young people, from children and infants. When a care home is built a new nursery could be sited in the same building, sharing a garden, a pond – a nursery where the staff of the care home can leave their children safely while they work, where children can fill the bird feeders or draw pictures of buses and spacemen for the walls.

We are all apprentice old people. Things that work well for people who are older tend also to make things better for everyone. Innovative, comfortable housing with minimal heating bills is something that is good not only for an older couple eking out a fixed pension, but also for a family struggling on a low income. Hospital systems that require attendance on several different days for tests and another visit for results are just as much a headache for a patient who is in middle age and must negotiate time off work, or for a child who is missing school as they are for someone with diminishing sight who is no longer able to drive. Everybody benefits if we design the delivery of care so that it meets the needs of our oldest, least mobile, most complex patients, using technology to streamline investigations and common sense to replace unwanted appointments with phone calls or messages, and using clear language to discuss decisions. Public transport that is reliable and can be used by someone who needs a walking frame works for a young mother with a toddler and a pram. Green places in cities make us happy – I read with a grin of the 'hedonometer', which is not really a meter but a computer algorithm that surveys the words used in social media messages. The hedonometer discovers, of course, that the messages sent by those in parks and countryside are disproportionately laden with positive phrases. If we make such places accessible and safe for our oldest people, those green places are there upping the happiness quota for our children too.

At every level making things better for those who are very old, makes things better for all of us. And we can do it. We can fix our health information systems so that essential details are shared securely and reliably across organizations. We can embrace invention, the ingenuity that allows us to see our brother laugh, whether he is in

Australia or in the next street. We can harness technology that will help us travel to a talk, a meeting, a party. We can have delicate, honest conversations with those whom we love about our hopes and fears for ourselves and each other, and we can shift the power of choice towards those about whom choices are made. We can bring ourselves collectively to make bold and fair changes to social care, which will bring benefit not only to those who receive such care but also to those who deliver it. More emotionally rewarding jobs, better support, better training, better pay and conditions. In that photo in George's home of the seaside wheelchair-paddling event it is not only the recipients of the push who are having fun. The pair doing the pushing are teenagers perhaps, or in their early twenties, and their faces are lit by joy.

'I don't want to be a burden,' my friend Vivienne worries as she packs her notebook for the history society meeting. 'I want to be an asset.'

I think about her words as I read a King's Fund report, 'Unconventional Health and Care'. Its author, Ben Collins, has made an uplifting study of five organizations that are doing things differently. They're mostly focused on younger people who are hard-pressed, caught up in socially impoverished and chaotic situations. Phrases in the report chime because there's a common theme of unlocking potential, of perceiving value in lives where conventional vision sees only demand. One young woman explains how she does not want to be 'just a service user, there to take something'. She describes the workshops she attends, run by a mental health charity that involves the people it helps, encouraging them into roles as volunteers and leaders, as sources of creativity and solutions. She says, 'When I come here I am treated as somebody with something to offer. I have needs but I also have strengths and capabilities. I have things to give.'

Looking back over my years as a geriatrician, I know that my patients have been assets, that they have had 'things to give', because I have been the recipient of their gifts. I have been given a look, a letter, a pat on the hand. I've been given cherry liqueurs, a plush singing snowman, a bottle of elderflower wine. A compliment on my dress. An email that caused me to sit at my desk, tears streaming. A bunch of lilies, a card, a photograph of a woman, vivacious, dancing. A laugh, a smile, a painting of a parrot. Advice that there is baby sick on my shoulder, a hint that my skirt is tucked into my knickers. A kiss, a hug, a sugared almond. A tree, a book. A folded note that contains love as tangible as a pressed flower. I've been given an article about the healing power of crystals, a portfolio of poems, a hand-written account of a grim event in Burma in 1943. I've been gently, politely propositioned. I've been given terrible jokes, funny stories. Secrets. I have been given lesson after lesson by those with whom I have worked.

I'm at the community hospital and pass Kathleen's

door – Mrs Graham, who fell and has spent so long on her journey of uncertain recovery. She's still here, months later, with her appliqué sweatshirts and her tot of sherry, slowly, slowly getting better from her fractures of one leg and the other. An orange light is flashing above the door, a buzzer is sounding, and I knock and look in. Liv the nurse is in there with Kathleen and has pressed the bell for help, with her elbow, I think, because they've got themselves in a muddle, she and Kathleen, in moving between the bed and the chair and trying to get dressed. Kathleen has become momentarily over-whelmed and is standing, clinging to the turning frame, and Liv has her arm around Kathleen's back, holding her, reassuring her, but if Kathleen goes down now, it will be between the bed and the chair, so she needs to hang on, to regain her composure, and it's hurting. Her worse leg is hurting, I can tell, as her eyes are screwed tight and her hands holding that frame are white. But it only takes an extra hand on her other side, no support really, just a touch, and she finds strength and breathes, and Liv is able to turn the frame round a little so Kathleen will be able to sit back safely into her chair. Yet before that Liv says, 'Steady on, Kath. Keep standing a mo and let's get those drawers up.'

I look down at the garment Liv's talking about and they're magnificent, sturdy and definitely drawers – ivory fabric with wide interlocked seams.

'You'd need two people to fold those,' Liv teases Kathleen, who growls, 'Get away with you.'

We wriggle her underwear into place, and there's something of the covered wagon about that garment, something that speaks of a pioneering spirit, of indefatigability. I've been given lesson after lesson in courage.

I've been given countless lessons in hubris. I've made a penny-dropping, subtle and satisfying diagnosis, followed the same day by the shameful realization that, caught up in pride, I have delivered the bad news it represented clumsily and thoughtlessly. I've congratulated myself on spotting a rare drug side effect and gone on to write up the wrong dose of the alternative. I have been rewarded by seeing my patient improve on the new tablets I chose for her only to find that she hasn't taken any of them, being averse to pink tablets, her recovery entirely down to someone else's intervention. I've explained to Edna that she is going to die imminently, her thoracic aortic aneurysm incontrovertibly leaking in a manner incompatible with life, and have greeted her every six months for many years since in outpatients, where we discuss her seventeen grandchildren and adjust the doses of her eleven favourite medications. I've got so many things wrong.

I've been given lessons in bad behaviour. I've seen selfishness, greed and rudeness in my patients, together with alarming magnifications of lifelong traits of narcissism and control. I've met families who put their own concerns before those of someone whose life is coming to an end, who are unable to let go. A son who tells me, 'Lucy, I am not ready for my mother to die,' so that his mother must hold him and comfort him even as she is leaving life. I've been given enough information to work out why sometimes a family may not be as prepared to help their frail parent as others might expect, and have been given lessons that have taught me why there are those whose graves will be danced upon and deservedly so.

I have been given other lessons too – in loyalty. In London, still a trainee, I meet Boswell, who is determined to take Dora home in order that she might die there of the cancer that is eating her up. No matter that he is alone and thin and his bones creak as he stands. 'Her mother asked my mother to ask me to see her home safe from a dance. She was seventeen and I was nineteen, and I've been seeing her home safe ever since. No reason to stop now.'

Lessons in friendship: Barry comes to clinic with Gerald, who does not read or write, but Barry was on the bins with Gerald for years, and he tells me that he and the rest of the team look out for Gerald and always will, so one or the other of them will bring him to clinic as long as he needs to come, to which declaration Gerald does not reply, being overcome, but bangs his fist on his knee and wipes his eye with the back of his hand.

I have been given lessons in stoical humour. I meet Prudence, who had recently attended yet another funeral – another old friend gone – and there she had greeted Peter, whom she hadn't seen for some time, only to find that Peter looked at her in surprise, saying, 'Prue, I could have sworn I'd been to yours last year.'

I have been given lessons in ingenuity, determination, acceptance, grace. Lesson after lesson.

The matron of our community hospital forwarded me a letter from Mrs Longford, whose husband died suddenly while he was recovering from a fracture. I have the letter still, years later. In even, curlicued script she thanks the staff for their care and expresses concern for the young nurse who was with William when he became so quickly pale and was gone. Mrs Longford writes: *I tried to reassure her because for many months he had been saying he had had enough and wanted to die . . . I am very relieved that he did not suffer.* Her letter continues: *I am glad that my beloved, gentle, charming William, still with his untouched sense of humour, was a patient at your hospital. I do feel bereft now after sixty-four years of a good marriage, but I am glad I have outlived him. I am ninety-three years of age, but we had no children or surviving relatives, so I am pleased that he will not be alone in this life and is now at peace.*

I have read Mrs Longford's letter many times now, but every time my breath is caught by the selflessness of her wish that William should die first in order that he be not lonely – her own loneliness inconsequential.

I am on my way to a meeting and there's a programme on the car radio about the naming of ships – the presenter is entranced by the naval vessels of the Second World War, and he describes his favourites, their commissioning and crews, and their service. Many did not survive, were lost in the cause of freedom. Their names are irresistible. HMS *Ardent*, HMS *Courageous*. *Hasty* and *Dasher*. HMS *Formidable*, HMS *Success*. *Lively*, *Fearless* and *Intrepid*.

The names roll softly around in my mind as I listen and drive, and then, ahead, there are red brake lights stacked up and the road is closed, an accident, I guess, so I turn and try to find a different way. The time ticks by, and now I'm on a tiny road that I haven't been on before, and a short row of houses comes up on my right. I read the white painted metal sign screwed to the first house of the terrace and realize that this is where Kathleen lives, who spent so long in our community hospital and made it home a few months ago. I look at the clock and the meeting is halfway done now, so I stop the car and slam the door.

It's been a chilly day so far, despite being June, with rain overnight and a puddle where Kathleen's little gate is, so I step round the puddle and the front door looks unused and dusty, so I go round the back, the cream pebble-dash wall of the house to my left, and find the kitchen door. I knock and let myself in through a porch with an umbrella in a basket and a shelf of empty vases, a deep red glass one and a white china one and others, then into a living room, which has Kathleen's bed in it and a chair and Kathleen herself, who nods and says, 'Oh, it's you, come to check up on me.'

And I assure her I am not checking, just passing. We talk of this and that, and how are the carers, and how is she? It's comfortably warm for there's a bar heater on and there is a smell of toast from breakfast, and the little figurine, the polka-dot bikini girl, is dancing on the mantelpiece above the heater, and on top of the television the man with the wavy hair and the pipe in his teeth is still sailing his dinghy.

Kathleen shows me a picture of her great-grandson, all gappy grin in a taekwondo outfit, and I look around and notice the walking frame tucked beside her chair and Kathleen's slippers with dark blue woolly pom-poms, and the hospital bed with its air mattress and rails. A blousy apricot rose is moving in the wind outside, knocking at the window, and Kathleen is wearing her appliqué dog sweatshirt, and she taps her fingers on the table beside her chair, once, twice, and says, 'It's good. It's all good.'

Kathleen, HMS *Undaunted*.

*

You can read Ben Collins's report here:
https://www.kingsfund.org.uk/publications/unconven
tional-health-care#seeing-things-differently

Epilogue

Something has gone wrong with one of our COVID-19 testing machines. For two weeks or so, or maybe longer – no one seems quite sure – it has been spitting out wrong results. We know no test is perfect. We are used to false negative results, for many people who have COVID-19 do not produce a positive test – the virus is hiding deep in their lungs, out of reach of the swabs that we take from nose and throat, but the bigger picture (their chest X-ray, their blood results, their CT scan) shows barn-door COVID-19; it can't be anything else. But this time the machine has made the opposite mistake, detecting a virus that is not there in routine swabs taken from people who have come in with other problems – an overdose, a heart attack, a urine infection – and this doesn't sound like such a bad thing on the surface; perhaps it'll be nice to be able to say, 'You know, we thought you had the virus, but you don't.' And this may be OK, a relief for some, but others will have been harmed. Their treatment has been based on a wrong result – perhaps there is harm ongoing, an alternative diagnosis that must be sought, or an operation that should have happened but has not (because surgery in an infected person is risky), or a family is racked with guilt and blame, believing that one among them has carried the virus into the home of a person they have all undertaken to protect. Or a lonely person has left hospital even lonelier, going home to a period of unnecessary self-isolation. For many of those affected we cannot now discern whether their result was a false positive or was, in fact, correct. The harms will be many and various. I am outraged that this error has happened. On top of all the other vile facets of this dismal pandemic – its effects on young and old, its disgusting, disproportionate grip on those who are already disadvantaged – this feels like a twist too far. I am incandescent.

A meeting of senior staff has been urgently convened, and I am angry, so angry, so worried, as I try to recall the patients for whom I've cared over the last few weeks, and the medical director is trying to explain the timeline, how the fault was detected, but I am talking furiously, firing questions as he speaks. I can see his mouth moving behind his mask, but I cannot hear him, and I suddenly feel a touch on my arm, because Claire, our divisional manager, has leaned forward from behind me and rests her hand on my arm for a moment, and I stop talking. I start listening. The meeting continues. We learn what has happened. We discuss what is known, what we still need to know, and what can never be known. We work out how we can mitigate harms, what will be done to prevent some similar problem, and how we can explain these events and plans to our patients and their families.

After work I take the dog for a walk, and I think about

anger. I hate this virus. What is the right way to respond? How do we each move forward from this global experience of anger, fear and uncertainty? Claire's hand, which stopped me in our meeting, conveyed more than a warning – had her message been only that perhaps I would have remained simply angry. But that brief touch carried other meanings – it held sympathy for my rage and impatience, and a knowledge of shared values, of trust.

At our best, in the face of this challenge, we come together. Medical teams and research scientists pool their resources and energy. Vast multinational databases are set up, to gather the information we need to help us make decisions. We start learning so quickly, building up knowledge. We elucidate every atom of the virus's structure, study the techniques it uses to enter our bodies, probe its weaknesses. We discover how it spreads; we catalogue its symptoms, which are legion. We run trials, share knowledge of treatments that work and that don't. Respected journals drop their paywalls – now anyone can read an important study, can analyse how another team's results affect the work of their own.

Kate Bingham, chairwoman of the UK Vaccine Taskforce, is challenged to explain why Russia, accused of attempts to steal research, should still be granted access to any successful vaccine. She is firm. 'This is a global pandemic and this is not a case where we protect the UK and everything else goes away. We have a fundamental need to ensure that all people around the world who are at risk of COVID infection get vaccinated. It doesn't matter whether you're in Russia or Timbuktu, that is a global commitment that we, the UK, have made and need to continue to make.'

There is self-interest here – this country may be set in the silver sea, but we are no longer an island – yet Kate Bingham's statement is also about values, commitment, fairness. Success in the fight against such a disease depends on global collaboration.

I watch the dog race ahead of me along the river, and I think next about the response of individuals, of older people and their families. What can we each do when faced with this new situation, uncertain, threatened? I think back to the meeting in which I was so angry and fearful for our patients, and how it became clear that we had to gather information, check through each individual's circumstances – social, medical – to find the correct response. It was essential that we base our approach on as many facts as we could muster, and equally clear that we would have to make decisions despite frustrating uncertainties. And as I consider this, I think about the misunderstandings and misconceptions that have sprung up around this virus. I must tread so softly here, because these are subjects that not only have been politicized, downplayed by one faction or highlighted by another, but are also emotive and highly sensitive for individual families. Words can be misconstrued, motives misinterpreted. The situation evolves – what was true yesterday may no longer be true tomorrow, good advice becomes outdated. I try to think, *What is good information, useful for my patients and their families to know?* I feel as if I'm walking through shifting sands, looking for islands of certainty, and those solid, important islands seem to me to be made of as much reliable information as we can gather, woven tightly together with an understanding of what we each desire from our lives.

Let us think first about what we know at present, about fear and fatality. We must be allowed to stand back for a moment, to counteract the impression given by night after night of TV coverage, of terrible – real and terrible – images from intensive care units, or of newspaper photo galleries, of victims young and old, but mostly old; a harrowing photograph of two women outside a care home, anguished, something dreadful has happened. These images have given so many of my patients and their families the impression that this illness is uniformly fatal for our oldest people, when it is not.

Dawn telephones the admission ward to ask about her father Eustace.

'Is it the virus?' she asks, and I tell her that there is a patch of infection on one of his lungs, a proper pneumonia, and that his COVID test is negative (and I am sure that result is correct, as there is no sign of COVID), and she exhales, a huge sigh of misplaced relief at it being 'only pneumonia', and I wonder how I can explain, whether I should explain (will it help Dawn to know?), that this pneumonia is, in Eugene's particular case, as likely to take his life as COVID-19 would have been – which is less likely than she thinks. In Dawn's mind

COVID is unsurvivable for her dad, but she has been given the wrong message. Even in his eighties, and even having become unwell enough to be hospitalized, Eugene would have a very reasonable chance of survival. This is important, partly because the fear generated by this virus is bad enough when the facts are straight. As I write, the evidence suggests that around 20% of people in their eighties or nineties who contract this virus will succumb to it. That is a huge number of people. However, four in five will survive, of whom most will not even need hospital treatment. These facts are also important because many older people have been given the wrong impression that should they become very ill with COVID-19 – ill enough to need oxygen, say – they are inevitably going to die, and that, therefore, the best thing to do is to stay put at home. There are some – not Eugene, who has few medical problems, and played bowls until lockdown, but others, closer already to the end of their lives for other reasons – for whom COVID-19 is indeed very likely to be a final illness, whatever supportive treatment is given, and they will not benefit from being bundled into an ambulance. And there are others too who will choose not to come to hospital, even when they know that they could benefit from hospital treatment in terms of living longer; they have decided that they don't want that option. The fact that many older people survive COVID-19 does not trivialize this illness nor detract from the level of suffering and loss it brings. But it is not fair for older people and their families to be given the impression that they should avoid attending hospital for treatment for this virus – or indeed for other unrelated illnesses, because otherwise many people will suffer unnecessarily, both *of* COVID and *because* of it.

The virus has thrown into focus many aspects of getting older that we have previously chosen to view only as if through milky glass. This new experience highlights the need for honesty, for sharing knowledge and being truthful about what is not known. In addition, it has held a magnifying lens over the need to talk openly about what is important to each of us, what matters most.

Mr Perez frowns, struggling to catch my words. His right hand, bony and bruised, moves to touch the oxygen tubing where the soft plastic prongs enter his nose; his left hand lies on the pale blue blanket, a gold watch sitting among the dark hairs at his wrist. His index finger is held by the oximeter. He has big coffee-coloured freckles on his smooth head. Fantastic eyebrows. Hearing aids.

'You look a bit better!' I shout from behind my mask, the words warming the air under my eyes, but he shakes his head, and I can't tell whether he cannot hear or whether he doesn't believe me, and so I give a thumbs up, both thumbs, and smile as widely as I can so that he might see my eyes crinkle above the mask, but Mr Perez tilts his head down and drops his eyes. So tired and scared.

In fact, he really is getting better, and I would like him to know that – to see what we can see, the improvement in his oxygen levels, the resolution of his blood results.

I'd like to talk to him about getting out of bed and having something to eat – what would he like? – and about his daughters, who have phoned again and are willing him to recover. I'd like to have a conversation too, handled as carefully as the fine, friable pages of a very old text, to make sure that Mr Perez knows about the plans we made with those daughters, and that he is in agreement with those plans. And this will be difficult, for it is more than simply my face mask that is obscuring our conversation.

David Oliver is a past president of the British Geriatrics Society, and for several years was the UK's National Clinical Director for Older People's Services. For one happy, busy year, we trained together in London, and I have met few people so single-minded in their pursuit of a better life for older people. Alongside his work as a geriatrician, he writes truthfully and with passion, challenging ageism and campaigning for improved services in health and social care, for more understanding of the joys and challenges of long lives. David knows what he is talking about, and in a *BMJ* article published in May 2020 he talks about old news. He writes, 'It's really struck me that many issues that were already clear to health professionals before the pandemic have now become news, when previously they struggled for attention outside specialist healthcare publications.'

David observes that problems were repeatedly highlighted by organizations familiar with health policy, but were largely ignored in mainstream media: the lack of pandemic preparedness, the UK's relative scarcity of acute and intensive care beds, endemic problems with social care and the disjunction of care homes from any consistent support by local NHS services. He notes how these issues have suddenly been propelled to the front page as the pandemic has unfolded. For many who are concerned with the well-being of older people this grim virus has shone some welcome light, presenting us with an opportunity to rethink, to change.

Yet alongside this, David is concerned. He explains how, before the pandemic, many elements of good practice were already in place, or were on a road towards becoming established. He says, 'Already it was a good idea to discuss resuscitation with patients and families and to have more structured, person-centred plans . . . to improve end-of-life care and avoid overmedicalization of natural dying.'

He explains that it was already right, before COVID, that medical teams should try to avoid sending someone very frail from their care home into the bewildering environment of the acute hospital, unless that person could both benefit from hospital treatment and wished to receive it. It was already right, he says, that we should try to provide as much treatment as we can, including palliative care when needed, in someone's familiar environment. David knows, as many older people and their families know, that older people can be harmed as well as helped by even the best-intentioned hospital treatment.

His article also tackles one of the subjects that has become most sensitive, that of ICU beds, of ventilators, and he outlines how teams have always made decisions about admission to ICU (which is completely separate from decisions about admission to hospital) based on increasingly sophisticated assessments of the patient's ability to benefit, using evidence-based scoring systems that go well beyond crude chronological age or subject-ive judgements about disability or quality of life. He explains how this is – was already – the right thing to do, to ensure that our patients are not subjected to treat-ments from which they cannot benefit.

And yet a narrative is developing in parts of the media that it is somehow bad, even scandalous, that these things – making advance care plans, being cautious about sending people to ICU – should be happening. David worries, 'Things that were already essentially good and often mainstream practice before the pan-demic are now presented as bad.'

How is it that we have generated two opposing narra-tives about the delicate conversations and decisions demanded by our long, long lives? I think about Mr Perez and his daughters, and how difficult it is for them to be confident that we are working together, to feel that their values and mine are aligned. Even before COVID, with all four of us sitting together, unmasked, with every opportunity for me to detect the tiniest signals of dis-tress, these conversations can go awry.

I have read those narratives, those angry sad stories, and I know they are real. They have common themes – of a conversation broached without warning, or even a form arriving in the post; a telephone call; an unfamiliar stranger who seems intent on one goal, the agreement of a DNAR order; an advance care plan found in a suitcase on returning from hospital. There's a constant under-current, a suggestion that a life isn't valued, that resources are limited. This reporting is not wilfully malign or obstructive; it reflects real interactions that, for all sorts of different reasons, have been insensitive, panicky, thoughtless. Bad conversations about these sensitive subjects existed before COVID, but the pandemic has accelerated them – it has come on us in a rush, with its fear and urgency, and we are ill prepared, on both sides of these conversations. Patients, families, journalists – all deserve better knowledge of what is being discussed: realistic facts, sensitively shared. Others – doctors, nurses – need a better appreciation of just how delicate, how tender, these discussions are for those whom they concern. Yet now, more than ever, we need to have these conversations, because when we get them right they are not about having something taken away, being denied life. They are instead a gift, an opportunity to talk about hopes and fears, a time for honesty and kindness.

How do we respond to the pandemic as a society? I think about lockdown, about isolation, and am in turmoil.

I listen to one of the carers from the home where Marjorie, who has fallen and broken her pelvis, lives. Linda explains how Marjorie has been deteriorating since the lockdown, less willing to walk, leaving her food. 'She was a cheery little soul,' says Linda, 'but she's just gone sort of . . . quiet. I think it's because of Bill. He used to visit come wind or shine. I think he was a little bit of heaven for her every day.'

I listen to Shirley. I am doing a phone clinic, and Kenneth is on the list. Shirley has woken him to speak to me, but he is muddled and cannot hear well. 'It's the doctor, Ken,' I hear her say. 'The doctor. No, that's no good, hold it closer.' And I hear Ken grumbling, and Shirley has taken up the phone again, and she and I talk about how things are, and Shirley says, 'I like this lockdown. I feel better shopping, because I was always worried before, with Ken's chest, that I would catch something in the shop and give it to him, and now everyone's being careful, and I feel safer now than I did before. It suits us.'

I listen to Jane, an old friend of Mum's; they go way back. 'It's very dull,' she says, and she will say no more, because she never, ever complains, despite being alone, and we talk instead of a foal in a field.

Gordon tells me, 'I'd take my chances,' but he hasn't, this is just talk, for Gordon has obeyed the rules, with Rita doing his shopping and leaving it on the doorstep.

There is a letter in the paper. 'I do not want to go on being alive, if I am not allowed to go on living.'

I ask patients, families, friends, colleagues. What is the way forward? How do we balance the potentially lethal effects of isolation with the need to control the potentially lethal virus? There are frowns and shrugs, and conversations that go round and round. Mention is made of the war years, 'We got through that,' but I look at the big posters in Tesco, 'Together, we can do this', which make me smile, except that so many older people are not 'together' – they are apart.

I look back at the last chapter – what should have been the last chapter – and its call for inclusivity, for care homes with kindergartens, and I wonder how unrealistic is that now, how naive? I read articles that demand selective, prolonged separation from the rest of society for 'the elderly' (I note the collective noun) – one in the *Economist*, and another in a journal of medical ethics. The latter is written by a man who is a professor of ethics, who I think should know better, until I look up his views on some other subjects and I realize that his ethical framework differs from my own. His is founded in utility, and leaves no room for the imperfect, the beautifully irrational, the heart swell of the human.

I do not hold either with those who would simply party on, who say we should just get it over with, let millions die. It is true that many of those who die of COVID-19 are very close to the end of their lives in any case (and these COVID deaths in the frailest are peaceful, not frightening), but many too are people, including very old people, who were not expecting to meet such an ending so soon, had other plans, lives to be getting on with.

I believe we can do better than either of those extremes. I do not accept – I do not think most of us believe – that older people are simply some inconvenient 'other' to be locked away. When we pause for a moment we recognize that older people are people right now, and ourselves tomorrow.

Equally we share a desire to protect. Gordon announces his plan to 'take his chances', but he doesn't – not because he is afraid (nothing much scares Gordon), but because he does not want to take someone else's chances alongside his own. But as well as being concerned for one another, we are resourceful, innovative and flexible. We will work out how we can restore freedoms bit by bit, and we shall have to be prepared for disappointments as ground will be lost before it is regained. We will search for a vaccine, but at the same time we will learn how to live with this virus. Being treated 'equally' does not mean being treated 'the same', and we are already gathering the knowledge we need in order to quantify risks for each individual, and can combine this with local knowledge of the prevalence of infection, and with our growing understanding of measures that keep us safe, even while we are close to other people. We will each have to decide what we do about risk. We shall have to think about what matters most, and that will require us to talk about what it means to be old, which, in fact, is just the same as what it means to be human.

At the height of lockdown I received letters and emails from a couple in their eighties, the dearest friends of my parents. They have known me since I was a baby, and their messages abound with energy and encouragement, but also with yearning.

The grandchildren – how I long for a cuddle, I read. *What we want is friends round our table, and lots of elbows on it.*

Oh, how I want my elbows on that table! I want to hear chatter, to watch someone leaning forward to emphasize a tale. To see arms thrown upwards in laughter, and to catch the expression of a quiet person who is listening. I want to stand up and splash wine into the glasses of friends, and spoon buttered potatoes from a huge saucepan.

Now more than ever the time has come for conversation, for honesty about the facts of getting older. For making plans together, so our wishes can be known and respected. For a reassessment of our society's structure, so that everyone – everyone – can live their lives to the fullest.

In a book by Michael Mayne, *The Enduring Melody*, written while he was very ill and knew that he did not have long to live, he describes a line of Shakespeare from the end of *The Tempest*, when the ageing Prospero swears that from now on 'every third thought shall be my grave'. Which, comments the American author John Updike, 'leaves two other thoughts to entertain above the ground: love one another, and seize the day'.

I have noticed something while writing this book, which is that each time someone has asked what it is about and I say it is about getting older, and the things we don't want to talk about, they smile. They always smile. The smiles may be happy, or anxious, or even regretful, but they are always present, and people say, 'That's a good subject. We should talk about that.'

Acknowledgements

THANK YOU to my colleagues, who supported my sabbatical without a murmur, and to geriatricians throughout my career from whom I have learned – thank you to Shah, Gerry, Fiona; to Mike and Kevin; particularly to Sheena – a grateful hug – and to Celia and Gucharan; to Adrian, Tony and Finbarr; to Mary, Paul, Tarun, Simon, Rachel, Anita, Sarah, Nahida, Tara, Matt and Ravi, and especially to Peter and Vikky. I could never have hoped for so much laughter. Thank you to Shelagh O'Riordan, Trisha Elliott and Emily Henderson for early reading and kind words from afar, and to our trainees Ella Sherman and Kirsty Nelson-Smith for insightful comments, and to Ella Burden, Camilla Paget and Hamish Macdonald for their work on resus outcomes. Thank you to Sandy, Lindsey, Kyra, David, Jenny, Emma and others in the Question Writing Group, passionate about education. To Zoe Wyrko and Jacqueline Close for their thoughts about care homes and falls respectively, and to Nick Warner and Mark Upton for their superb insights into dementia, and to David Oliver for inspiration and courage.

Thank you to Zoe Fritz and Catherine Baldock for advice about the ReSPECT documentation, and to Marion Jones from the NHS blood and transplant team, and to Tamsin Leeper and Emma Gray for accurate words about the legal aspects of getting older, and to Sarah Orr and the team at the GMC for their careful reading of several chapters.

Thank you to so many hardworking, wise and warm-hearted nurses, among whom shine Maggie and Sally, Julia, Jane, Pauline, Viv, Mary, Annie, Elaine, James, Claire, Caroline, Robert, Mel, Alex, Helen and many more. Thank you to Julie Jones, Wendy Burman, Stuart Walker and Peter Lewis for making my sabbatical happen, among other good things; to HCAs like Dot, and Maggie, Lianne and Sammy, who laugh, and work, and care day after day; to physios and their assistants like Clare, Barry, Jenny, Chris, Sarah and John; and OTs and their assistants too, like Eleanor, Jim, Karen and Sian; and to social workers like Gill and Renu; to Colleen, Heulwyn and Ellie for the power of their listening to people who needed to talk. To Lindy, Andrea, Karen, Kelly, Sheena, Amanda, Vicky and the rest of the office team for Berocca, biscuits and problem-solving. Thank you to members past and present of the Clinical Ethics Committee, thoughtful and unafraid, and to Sarah Bridges, Anna Baverstock and Debbie Stalker, the best ever appraisers.

A huge thank-you to countless students and doctors in training, who have shared long hours, dodgy sandwiches, Mellow Birds coffee, learning and laughter, and who make me listen when I've stopped listening, and who so often have caught me when I've fallen.

Thank you to Kathryn Mannix for permission to use her beautiful words about dying, and to Elaine Miller, gusset gripper, for allowing me to use her words too, and for making me laugh enough to test my own pelvic floor. To Carol-Ann, Siobhan and the ever-obliging library team and to George Coxon and Ben Collins, who think about the value of undervalued people.

Thank you to my dear aunt Mary Crossley for liking what she read, and to Vicky, Hugo, Josh and Suze, for patient listening over many years, and to Mary Fryer, Jane Gotto, Margaret Turner, Annie Taylor, Isabel Oliver, Nigel Riglar, Robin Littman, Paul and Elizabeth Heim, and Johnny and Ann Tusa, for gentle goodwill, sound advice and useful words. Thank you to my terrific friends, Charlotte, Katharine, Lou, Mary, Miranda, Pip, Selina and Zanna, for conviviality and joy, and to Clodagh de Jode who always believed in this project.

Thank you to the remarkable Beth Miller, https://www.bethmiller.co.uk, for knowledgeable and accurate early shepherding, and to Sam Knowles for sending me in Beth's direction.

Huge thanks to the incomparable Michael Joseph / Penguin Random House team: to Clare Parker, Ella Watkins, Emma Henderson and Katie Williams, and special thanks to Colin Brush for the perfect title, and to Lauren Wakefield, Lee Motley and Christophe Jacques for the cover.

Thank you to Tess Stimson for stalwart friendship and a very good email, and to Louise Moore, vibrant and passionate, who gave me the (incredible, ecstatic) opportunity to write this book. Thank you to dear Ariel Pakier for such kind, thoughtful and clever editorial direction, and to my agent Cathryn Summerhayes, wide smile, who makes me happy.

Thank you to Gail, and to Sash and Lucy, for their immense generosity in providing their homes – two perfect, bird-filled hiding places.

Thank you to my unique patients and to their families, friends and carers. I think especially and with profound gratitude of Christine, Michael, Mavis, another Mavis, and Moira, and a very small determined woman in a red coat with gold buttons, whose stories are not told.

Thank you to my family, who mean the world to me: to Flora, Ben and Letty; and to Giles, patient, unexpected, loving. Loved.

Index